NEW ENLARGED EDITION

Arthritis and Common Sense

by

DAN DALE ALEXANDER

ILLUSTRATED   **WITH MENUS**

WITKOWER PRESS
INCORPORATED
Hartford, Connecticut

TO EDITH

Whose help, encouragement and patience made this book possible. As my wife, she has endured loneliness—while I worked through the long nights in laboratories, through thousands of tests, and through the long years of duty in hospitals. Still alone, she waited patiently while I traveled across America four times to do arthritic research in hundreds of cities.

As my helpmate, she has recorded facts, typed endless reports, and she even tested personally the actual menus and dietary plans. From her schooling in art, she drew the illustrations found throughout this book. In addition to all this, she has somehow found time to raise our children . . . has made for all of us a healthy, happy home.

So . . . to Edith . . . I dedicate this volume.

Table of Contents

Preface   v

Foreword   1

I   Why and How This Book Was Written ...   5

II   A Preview of What's to Come   11

III   Understand All Arthritis—Recognize Your Own Type   17

IV   Combat Dryness in the Joint Linings and Cartilage   35

V   Faulty Diet Can Cause Arthritis   45

VI   The Right Foods—To Help Gain Relief ..   51

VII   Fruits and Their Effect on Bodily Oils ...   67

VIII   Modern Beverages—A Help or Hindrance?   79

IX   About Our Habits . . . Eating, Drinking, Smoking   87

X   Do Charts on Health Have Any Value? ...   91

XI   Shift the Liquids in Your Diet   97

XII   Drinking Water—a Curse or a Blessing?...   109

XIII   Acids in Food Lead to Sensitivity   121

XIV   Avoid Foods with the Wrong Oils   127

XV   Menus . . . Day by Day List of Correct Meals   133

XVI   Can Vitamins Speed Relief?   153

XVII   Cod Liver Oil Is a Key Weapon   159

XVIII   Your Liver Can Cheat You   171

XIX   How Constipation Affects Arthritics   183

XX   Cortisone Can Help, But Not Cure   203

XXI   Superstitions and False Remedies   213

XXII   The Rate of Recovery   229

XXIII   The Answer to Your Key Questions   235

XXIV   What the Future Holds for Arthritics   241

PREFACE

Since the first and second editions of this book were published, a great deal has happened to me, the author.

Now, as I write this third edition—as I add new facts, additional findings and minor changes to clarify medical language for readers—I would like to report on how this book has already helped many people gain relief from their arthritis.

During the past year, thousands of letters have been sent to me from all parts of the country. Victims of arthritis—throughout America—have tried my dietary plan, as outlined in these pages. They write that their pain and the swelling in their joints disappear . . . and they have been able to resume normal and happy lives.

Receiving such letters has become the greatest experience of my life. For fourteen long years, I have done research work and intensive studying to find the answer to arthritis . . . and, now, these letters make all my efforts seem worth while.

To know that this book is helping to relieve suffering is the most satisfying reward any writer could ask.

As I review the history of this book, let me speak frankly. Naturally, all the comments about this manuscript have not been favorable. With any new idea, there are always expressions pro and con, at first.

Many physicians have recommended my book to their patients, others have attacked my discoveries. Right now, doctors in New England, the Mid-West and in California are treating arthritics under the methods I outlined in this book. Test cases, under medical supervision, are continuing daily.

The medical profession is entitled to question, experiment with and analyze the facts in this book. We expected that doctors would, and we welcome their tests and comments.

This is a new method for treating arthritis. And, here is the most important fact . . . *People are obtaining relief from arthritic pains and symptoms* through my dietary regime. The plan works, letters pouring in to me prove the results! More and more doctors are adopting the program.

So, as a preface, let me describe what you will find in these pages. . . .

This book tells about arthritis, its causes, effects and a safe and sane approach toward its relief.

You will find in these pages a list of menus, a day by day breakdown of meals I recommend for arthritics . . . a plan of good eating for an entire week. And we have added certain illustrations and new chapters to present a more complete picture of my discoveries.

The language in this book is simple, easy to read. The manuscript is intended mainly for the person with little or no medical knowledge—to give a clear explanation of his affliction.

Anyone seeking an over-night cure should look to the "wonder drugs" now being over-publicized. However, the "quick cure" claimed through drugs may prove to be temporary—and the drug treatments may have to be stopped to prevent different complications.

Let us draw a comparison with diabetes. Instead of using drugs, medical science is now turning back to the diet to control this metabolic disorder. Now, after many years of using hormonal insulin, treatment by diet is becoming an accepted method.

The same development is due in regard to arthritis. Before many years, medical science will turn back to diet to treat arthritis.

Arthritis generally begins slowly and is often due to a combination of dietary mistakes. Primarily the "basic" mistakes leading to arthritis are:

(a) *Key nutritional oils* in the daily meals are either missing, or if present, are not assimilated properly. Frequently, it takes several to many years of poor food choice and/or poor eating habits to lead to an arthritic condition.

(b) On the other hand—the correct nutritional oils "can be" in many of the daily meals and even accomplish their proper lubricating job. *BUT IN OTHER MEALS,* "oil deteriorating liquids or other detrimental, devitalized foods" can still undermine "the good" of previous meals *"ALREADY" PROPERLY ASSIMILATED.*

Gradually— *the absence, confliction or deterioration of certain key nutritional dietary oils lead to a joint problem susceptibility. Then the lesser dietary mistakes, of which there are many, begin to take effect.*

In due time—*depending on the structure and pattern of the dietary mistakes—A PARTICULAR KIND OF ARTHRITIS SETS IN . . . . . be it osteo arthritis, rheumatoid or gouty arthritis.*

This book tells the proper diet, the selection and rotation of food, plus a dietetic therapy, so that more of the correct oils in your food can serve the joints. It also shows how these oils can stimulate your adrenal glands—to successfully combat arthritis.

Your own doctor is the man to see to determine whether you have arthritis. Visit your physician for a diagnosis, to decide if you have this dread disease. And I have always recommended that arthritics return to their doctors for periodic check-ups, to chart the progress of their recovery.

Meanwhile, however, this book maintains that it is possible for you to gain relief through simple diet controls. In these pages you will find a common sense approach for coping with arthritis right in your own home.

May this third edition of my book lead you to better health.

Miamis Road   DAN DALE ALEXANDER
West Hartford, Connecticut

FOREWORD

As a doctor, I feel that this book is an important contribution toward finding the answer to arthritis.

Dan Dale Alexander's methods and dietary approach have already gained excellent results for victims of this disease.

I have seen a former patient of mine who, because of arthritis, had reached the condition where she was unable to open her mouth enough to eat properly. When she followed the diet outlined by Mr. Alexander—and added proper oils to her system by his method—a miracle happened. Her improvement was markedly advanced.

In another case, I have talked with a mother and I have seen her ten-year-old child who was afflicted with arthritis. For five years the child had been given every treatment known to medical science to try to relieve her rheumatoid arthritis. Everything had been tried—including concentrated preparations of oil—but the patient responded only when her diet was corrected and the oil in its pure form was administered by the method revealed in this book.

The patient is now free of arthritis advancement and is 90% improved.

The victims described above are typical, and

1

they had serious cases of arthritis. For the majority of arthritics—whose cases are only in the early and moderately advanced stages—this book can hold even more benefit!

In addition to the special diet which the author explains in the book, he also advocates the use of cod liver oil. My own experience with cod liver oil dates back 50 years, when I started using it with my patients in the treatment of tuberculosis. Medical literature is full of accounts of its use as a folk remedy several hundred years back in the treatment of rheumatism and arthritis.

It has remained for Mr. Alexander to unlock its great value by a new and unique method of administration.

Simultaneously while taking the cod liver oil for joint relief, the dry skin is nourished and takes on lustre; the dry scalp and hair are corrected—the hair takes on a shine; the nails stop splitting, and the ears begin to secrete a normal amount of ear wax. The sedimentation rate returns to normal.

The vitamin A in cod liver oil benefits the eyes as well as the skin, but it remains for the small amount of vitamin D in the oil to give the oil its therapeutic quality for arthritics.

The vitamin D makes cod liver oil a steroid product of tremendous importance in combating both rheumatoid and osteo arthritis, because its dual action is on the adrenal glands and the syno-

vial membrane (joint linings), thus arresting cartilage degeneration.

Medical literature says arthritis is a constitutional disease. Here, at last—in this book—is a
logical, systemic approach. The entire body benefits from the Alexander diet, which emphasizes the
proper sequence of eating foods. (A new idea on
dieting for health.)

There is no remedy in use today which will
produce the feeling of well-being, the appearance
of health, that I have seen follow the use of Alexander's method.

As a doctor, I read and agreed with the second
edition of Alexander's book. He has spent years of
scientific research to develop his discoveries, and it
has been a privilege for me to write this foreword
for his Third Edition of *Arthritis and Common
Sense*.

H. E. Kirschner, M.D.

August 7, 1953
Monrovia, California

Chapter I

Why and How This Book Was Written

To know arthritis, you must experience it. As I have. I have felt the pain personally. During the course of my laboratory experiments, I purposely developed an arthritic condition within my own body. You don't have to tell me that this disease "hurts." It does, terribly.

Even worse than my own feelings, I have had a serious case of arthritis strike in my family. My mother became wracked with arthritic pains, and I saw her suffer for 10 long years. I have lived with this disease—and I know the damage it can do within a family and home.

For all these reasons, I decided to devote my life to fighting this illness. To tell you what I've done in the field of arthritis, and how I've done it, let's go back to the beginning. Back to a day in 1929.

It was then, 24 years ago, that I remember the onset of my mother's first aches and pains. They started in her shoulders, and at that time I heard her ailment called "rheumatism." My youth and inexperience left me in a sympathetic state, wanting to help, but unable to do so.

Back in those days, the use of heat was suggested and the usual electric pad was bought. So were salves, ointments and soothing oils of wintergreen. The relief felt from the externally applied heat was only temporary. The other medications did nothing.

Since the small town in which we lived did not have a specialist, mother went to a larger city to seek help. On the advice of a doctor there, she had X-rays taken. From the pictures came his decision as to a cure: tooth extraction. Every last tooth came out. The dentist was merely following orders, but I can still see the disappointment in my mother's face. Her teeth had been taken, but the arthritic pains remained as bad as ever.

Years later, I was to read many reports on how tooth extraction to cure arthritis was rampant in the 1930's. Not only teeth, but also tonsils and the appendix were considered to be the offenders—and were removed surgically. How many countless thousands of people with rheumatism sacrificed their teeth in this futile war against the disease!

Science has since established that arthritis is not infectious and that surgery on such organs is not necessary. Tooth extraction as a "cure" is frowned upon today. But every night the dish of water in which mother's teeth reposed reminded me of the foolishness to which she had been subjected.

For the next six years, she accepted her painful shoulders. Then, she went out again and sought medical advice. This time my mother brought home some little white tablets. No one knew what they were. But she took them whenever she had extreme pain. No improvement.

By 1940, mother's condition was changing rapidly. In addition to her earlier rheumatism, her hands were now swollen. She could no longer be the mistress of her kitchen. What she enjoyed doing most, her cooking, became a trial. She could not open and close her hands. Stairs were an effort to climb, because her knees were bothering her so much. The family never heard her complain. She suffered in silence.

To watch the agony of a loved one is heartbreaking. To know that there is practically nothing one can do about it is maddening. For every disease that exists, there is an army of men working to learn its cause and its cure. Each contribution, be it large or small, is of the utmost value. So, the thought occurred to me that perhaps I, too, could give something—to help my mother and all others like her who were afflicted.

Since that moment of realization I have been dedicated to this cause. My whole lifetime has been spent searching for the answer to arthritis.

To enumerate the countless experiments, the hours, days, and years of study and research . . . to tell how many authorities I have questioned on the subject, my making coast-to-coast trips . . . to describe the laboratory tests I made would fill a book. It has. This book. The book you are now reading will tell the whole story.

I will say, however, that before I subjected others to my discoveries, I applied my new theories to myself. By diet and other means I created arthritic symptoms and pains in my own bodily joints. I did this so that I could actually know the suffering an arthritic bears. So that I could better understand this affliction and its effects.

Later, by using my own discoveries, I defeated my "arthritis" and regained full health!

As added experience I attended Trinity College, studying the pre-medical course . . . and then pursued my search in the laboratories of the Air Force General Hospital, San Antonio, Texas. After taking courses at Columbia University, I collaborated for two years with an orthopedic surgeon in New York City and saw my work being carried on under medical supervision. The next three years were spent in the laboratories of a Connecticut hospital. There were so many questions to be answered, so many answers to be questioned.

The summary of my fourteen years' work is in this book. It is written for other mothers—and for all arthritics—to spare them untold miseries and perhaps a crippled or invalided body. This book is written for the medical profession, too. It has been read by scores of alert doctors who are interested in every new approach to arthritis. Many professional men already agree on its value.

Whether you are reading this book because of your own arthritis—or because one of your loved ones has it—it is my fervent prayer that this contribution of mine may be the missing piece to solve your arthritic problem.

MORE AND MORE CASES OF ARTHRITIS . . .

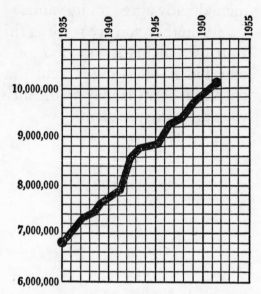

In recent years, the number of arthritics has been **INCREASING BY THE MIL-LIONS!**

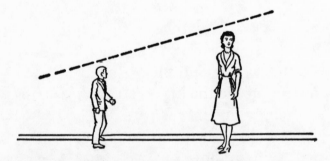

THREE TIMES AS MANY WOMEN BECOME VICTIMS OF ARTHRITIS

Female arthritics outnumber the men—THREE TO ONE!

Chapter II

A Preview of What's to Come

It is supposed to be bad writing to reveal the plot of a story before you tell it. However, I am now going to give you a "preview" of what you will find in this book. I will now reveal, in advance, what the chapters will contain.

My reasons for this unusual procedure are two: First, you may be particularly interested in some certain type of arthritis, or some drug, or some special treatment. By giving you an advance guide on how this book was put together, you can thumb the pages and find the chapter which you most want to read. You can jump directly to whatever phase concerns you. (Naturally, we hope you will read the entire book, because you'll gain the most benefit that way . . . but, meanwhile, use this chapter as a reference to the highlights which are ahead.)

Secondly, in this "preview" you are now reading, I will show the logic behind my discoveries. You will see how I arrived at various conclusions about arthritis. How my dietary plan grew, step by step, logically and based on proven medical facts.

I will admit that a chapter like this is a strange

thing for an author to do—revealing the "plot" too soon. However, perhaps I will be forgiven, because I am not really an author. I have never pretended to be a "literary" person. On the contrary, this is my first attempt to write a manuscript.

You see, for most of the past 14 years I have been a laboratory technician, working with test-tubes and scientific equipment. Not with words.

This may be an advantage to you, the reader. Because instead of filling this book with "literary" adjectives, I will state my findings in plain ordinary English. In fact, I have made a special effort to keep the language simple and understandable. I have purposely removed all medical terminology and "scientific-type" words from the text.

There is one word, however, which we all must understand here at the outset. That word is "ARTHRITIS." Let's examine it closely.

The prefix "arth" means "joint." The suffix "itis" is defined as "inflammation." Therefore, compounded, "arthritis" means "inflammation of the joint." What causes this inflammation? What causes arthritis?

Friction causes bodily joints to become inflamed. If the oils in your body dry out, the joints begin to creak. The joints rub against each other, and a grinding action sets in. The bony structure becomes damaged—and the whole area becomes swollen and inflamed!

There, stated simply, is the basis of my work. I set out to find a way to <u>lubricate</u> the joints and to reduce friction.

After years of scientific tests—we tried soy bean oil, corn oil, peanut oil and hundreds of others—we discovered that only one type of oil would do the lubrication job. Vitamin D oil was the only answer.

(Why vitamin D oil helps arthritis is described in Chapters XVI, XVII, and at many other points throughout this book.)

Next, we found that diet and eating habits could add specific oils to your body to aid your drying joints. (See Chapters VI, VII, XIV and many other pages as you read through the book.)

To increase the flow of all oils, and to add more of vitamin D oil to your system, we then developed a series of special diets. What foods were best for arthritics. Actual menus are included later in the book, and I think you are going to be very surprised by what you read. The menus will be pleasant tasting and nutritious.

We are not going to tell you to go on a strict diet. We are not going to urge people to starve themselves, and will not recommend a long list of "unusual" or strange foods. To defeat your arthritis, it's not so much what you eat. It's the order in which you eat your foods. How to eat your food, and when.

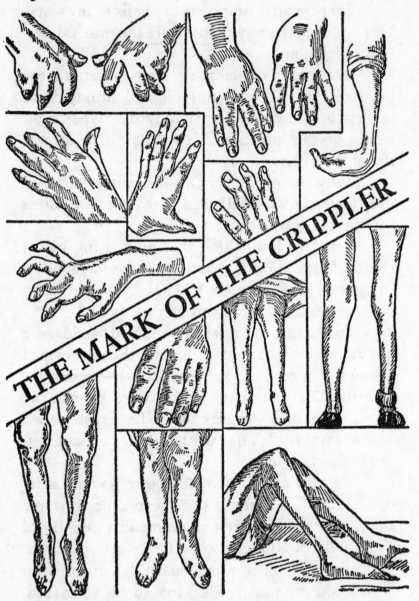

ARTHRITIS

**A Few of the Areas Where
This Affliction Strikes**

This book maintains that you can eat your way into arthritis—and you can eat your way out.

We shall deflate a great many rumors about arthritis, too. Expose them, and prove them false. (In Chapter XXI, for example.) Among them is the old tale about weather causing arthritis. Climate— winds, rain and sun—do not bring on your arthritis. Nor will weather cure the pains.

If geography had anything to do with this disease, why are there arthritics born and raised in sunny Florida as well as in the snow-clad regions of Montana? Do you realize that there are some 10,-000,000 victims of arthritis in the United States?

Think of it . . . ten million people suffering from some form of this ailment. This fact is proven by a survey conducted by the United States Government in 1951. Arthritis and "rheumatism" is on the increase daily. The toll has risen from approximately 6,850,000 victims, at the time of the last survey in 1935, to the current mark of ten million!

The results of this important survey by the Federal Government are available to you. For some startling and helpful information about arthritis, we suggest that you write for a copy of this report. It is entitled *Prevalence of Arthritis and Rheumatism in the United States,* and can be had by merely sending a nickel to the Superintendent of Documents, U. S. Government Printing Office, Washington 25, D.C.

So, as you can see, you are not alone in your arthritic pains and problems. Ten million of your neighbors are afflicted, too, and it is past time when we should do something to stop the spread of "the crippler."

As the first step, let's go on to the next page and learn all we can about ARTHRITIS. . . .

Chapter III

Understand All Arthritis—Recognize Your Own Type

Before we can learn how to recover from any disease, we must know exactly what the illness really is. As you probably realize, there are many types of arthritis, each with different symptoms, different areas of pain and different methods of relief.

Quite naturally, you are most interested in the type of arthritis which affects you. But the logic and facts in this book will make little sense to you unless you understand all forms of arthritis. Then, with a complete knowledge of the disease in general, you will be able to narrow down your own symptoms. You will be able to recognize which phase of arthritis concerns you most . . . so you can concentrate on your special kind and defeat it.

So, here, at the start of the book, let us examine arthritis as an overall problem. Let's investigate the two main types—osteo and rheumatoid arthritis—plus the other lesser known "brands." We will look at the illness in simple terms, without complicated medical language.

OSTEO ARTHRITIS—*Most Common of All*

More millions of people suffer from "osteo arthritis" than any other classification. We already know, from the last chapter, that the word "arthritis" means "inflammation of the joint." The word "osteo" comes from the Greek word "osteon," meaning "bone." Compounded, therefore, osteo arthritis can be defined as "inflammation of the bony part of the joint."

Your joints have many parts—membranes, cartilage, oil sacs, bones, etc. Osteo arthritis afflicts mainly the bone section, and so derives its name.

Osteo arthritis is known as a "wear and tear" disease. Overactivity in work or exercise can cause wearing out of the cushion of cartilage at the end of a bone. (Sometimes doctors also refer to "osteo" under the names of degenerative or hypertrophic arthritis.)

We maintain, however, that osteo arthritis is much more than just a question of bones simply wearing out. For every million persons who have this "wear and tear arthritis," there are twenty million people of the same age, doing the same type of work, who do not have the disease. Why? Because those who are well have better dietary habits!

In the *Journal of the American Medical Asso-*

ciation (July 2, 1949) Dr. E. F. Rosenberg reports that it is time to refute the belief that osteo arthritis comes from aging. As proof, this prominent Chicago doctor makes the following points:

1. Osteo arthritis of the fingers involves only the terminal joints. As the joints of the entire finger are used, why aren't the other joints affected?
2. Only one hip may become afflicted with osteo arthritis. Yet, through the years, both hips received the same amount of use.
3. Sedentary workers are often victims of osteo arthritis—without any mechanical or physical wear on their skeletal structure.

Where does osteo arthritis generally strike? Among men the most common joints affected are the knees, feet and spine. In women, it generally involves the fingers, hands, then the knees and spine. In other words, the parts of the body which do the work feel it first.

If you suffer from this ailment, you at least have plenty of company. More than 70% of the American population contracts some degree of osteo arthritis by the time they reach 55 years of age!

And this terrible toll has been high for centuries, back to the beginning of time.

Osteo Arthritis—as Old as the Hills!

This disease began more than 100,000,000 years ago. Fossils of dinosaurs in museums today show that before these animals died, their joints wore out. Their bones rubbed against each other, and frayed in arthritic manner.

During the time of the Egyptians, Greeks and Romans, osteo arthritis flourished.

In prehistoric and Roman times, just like to-day every animal and human had one dietary fault in common. They all drank too much water with their meals. In Chapter XII, later in this book, we will discuss in detail how improper water-drinking habits lead to arthritis.

RHEUMATOID ARTHRITIS, *the Crippler*

The second type of arthritis which we should learn to recognize is the rheumatoid kind.

The derivation of the word *rheumatoid* gives us an accurate picture of the feeling it produces. The root "rheuma" is from the Greek word meaning "flowing," and implies pain. The suffix "toid" means "similar to." Compounded, we have: *"similar to flowing pain."*

Rheumatoid arthritis first affects the mem-brane near your joints, rather than the bones themselves. Later, when the disease becomes chronic, bones are often distended and crippling results. (In addition to calling your condition "rheumatoid," your doctor may use the term "atrophic" or "proliferative" arthritis.)

Rheumatoid arthritis only became known in recent generations. This disease is attacking not only the 50 to 90-year-old age groups, but the youth of America, as well. It strikes teenagers, young soldiers and airmen, and even two-year-old children.

Two questions immediately arise: "Can anything in our diet be responsible for the increase in rheumatoid arthritis?" "And what element in food causes young people to be susceptible?" These days, youngsters demand more and more SUGAR with their meals or in their "snacks."

Sugar Leads to Trouble

Our youth are caught in a growing fad for sweetened liquids. Orange juice for breakfast—fruit sugar. Sugar on cereals. Soda pop with lunch —sugar. Plus solid sugars in candy, starchy meals and rich desserts!

Sugar destroys lubricating oils in our bodies which are needed to fight arthritis. Excessive sugar also deteriorates the intestinal wall. Once degenerated, the intestinal wall lets sugar molecules be transmitted almost at random into the linings of your joints. There it burns out the oil in the joint lining.

We want to condemn this sugar action as strongly as possible. Arthritics must realize that sugar can attack your bodily oils, leave the linings in a wasting condition, subject to scar tissue. As the oils waste away under the influence of sugar, the tissue fluids gel and stiffening sets in. The next stage is from stiffness to becoming crippled.

This discussion about the serious dangers of sugar has been placed in this section of the book pertaining to rheumatoid arthritis. But, may we emphasize that sugar is wrong for all arthritics of all types.

Now, let us proceed to a third classification of the disease. . . .

GOUTY ARTHRITIS

Many people never realize that the ailment known as "gout" is actually a form of arthritis. Confined mostly to the feet, although it occasionally strikes the hands and ears, "gouty arthritis" consists mainly of deposits of uric acid which accumulate in soft tissues of your body.

These drops of uric acid are responsible for the birth of the word "gout." It comes from the Latin word "gutta," meaning "drop." Years ago the Egyptians, Greeks and Romans envisioned poisonous crystals coming from the blood, drop by drop, and being deposited in the big toe.

The deposits cause the toe to swell up like a balloon and become extremely painful. Sometimes the crystals concentrate themselves in the ear, finger or knee. These chalky deposits are uric acid crystals.

There have been at least three schools of thought as to what causes gouty arthritis. The blame is often placed on: 1) Wine or fermented beverages, 2) high purine diet, or 3) defects in digestion and assimilation.

Today, records in the United States show about 20 cases of gout among every 10,000 arthritics. In countries like France and Italy, there are 250 or more cases of gouty arthritis per 10,000. In India, a country of vegetarians and teetotalers, the rate is 700 per 10,000.

If we go back into history to the Egyptians, Greeks and Romans, we find that they had osteo arthritis, but a much higher rate of gouty arthritis. Perhaps it was because they did drink a great deal of wine with their meals.

Fifty years ago, more Americans favored wine with meals than is evident today. As our rate of wine-drinking declined, so did the percentage of gouty arthritis.

The high purine diet (too many sweetbreads, anchovies, sardines, liver, kidneys, brains, and meat extracts) complicates gouty arthritis. Gout victims, by cutting down on the nitrogen-rich meats, have been freed from pain temporarily but we believe, however, that it is what you drink with your diet that decides your rate of recovery.

Today the gouty arthritis percentage among Americans is declining but overseas it still stays high. There they favor quantities of wine and fermented beverages with their meals. This custom puts a double duty on the liver, requiring it to detoxify the wrong liquids while it tries at the same time to utilize the meal.

Other Rheumatic Conditions

We have now discussed the three main categories of arthritis—gouty, rheumatoid and osteo. These three types combined include 95% of all victims of arthritis. Your case probably falls into one of those three classifications.

In addition, however, your arthritis may be complicated because you are also a victim of other rheumatic ailments at the same time. Therefore, let us examine several of the most common rheumatic conditions which are closely related to arthritis. We should understand these, too.

BURSITIS. When you develop pain in your shoulder muscles and calcium is forming in the bursae (the pouch or sac), the bursae have run out of oil. You are eating wrong and you may also be overexercising. You have bursitis.

There are different ways in which the problem of bursitis is met. Sometimes the calcium is "chopped" up with the aid of a long needle under sterile conditions. The more sensible way would be to "correct poor eating habits" which frequently lead to calcium deposits. The dietary regime in this book has been found to be very effective in controlling bursitis.

NEURITIS. If the oil sheath which covers your nerves dries out, you have neuritis. Another way of saying it would be "rheumatism in your nerves." Oils in your food are supposed to keep the nerve coatings intact. But only certain kinds of oil can perform the task. (We will tell you which oils are best, later in this book in Chapter XIV.)

Years ago, neuritis was known as neuralgia. Sciatic neuritis generally means that the oil has been stripped from over the sciatic nerve.

MYOSITIS. Working hard means that you tax many muscles in your body. When muscles have no oil to lubricate them, friction occurs in the muscles. You then acquire myositis.

FIBROSITIS. When your connective tissue or fibres become inflamed, you have "fibrositis." Some experts claim this ailment is of mental origin. We suggest checking your diet, for a general lack of oils.

LUMBAGO. Often, lumbago (sacroiliac strain) is a forerunner of arthritis in the spinal column. Our body is warning us that we cannot run our motors without oil. We dry out and squeak on for years. Then what do we do? We apply mustard plasters or force ourselves to undergo X-ray treatments. Back stiffness means that your tissue fluids are gelling. Eat more oil-bearing foods.

Compare Your Body to an Automobile

In the paragraph above we stated that we "can't run our motors without oil." This applies to the "bodily motor" just as well as to the machinery in the family car. As you probably noticed, when we discussed each type of arthritis and all the rheumatic ailments, we kept mentioning the need for oil to aid recovery. To prove our point and make this fact completely clear, let's compare our human body to an automobile. We will find some very interesting parallels. . . .

Your car has "joints" too. Its smooth functioning depends upon a constant supply of lubricating oils to prevent friction. Once the oil has run dry in your automobile, a grinding effect sets in and the parts cannot possibly function without damage.

With "dry joints" after 20,000 miles of driving, the bearings of the car—and the fittings become "frayed" and worn out. No amount of grease or sprayed oil can ever repair the broken part. Adding oil at this late date will stop the friction. But the end of the joint will remain worn down.

When you take your automobile to a garage or a lubritorium, you are asking the garage attendant to "remove the arthritis" from your car. With grease and oil of varying consistencies, he can take away the joint friction from your squeaking vehicle.

By the same token, the joints of a human body are dependent upon the joint lining and the blood-stream for a constant supply of lubricating materials. Without obtaining oils from your daily diet, your joints will degenerate and break down.

It will be helpful for arthritics to know exactly what types of joints are involved in the disease. Here are the four main categories found in our bodies:

The ball and socket joint. A smooth, rounded head of bone fits into a cup-like socket of another bone, permitting motion in all directions. The shoulder and hips are examples of this type.

The saddle joint. Here the bones move in two directions. The spinal vertebrae are in this category.

The rotary joint. These can rotate about an axis, like a key in a door. The elbow is one rotary joint.

The hinge joint. This type moves in only one direction, like those in your knees.

Regardless of the type of joint, they are ALL surrounded by linings which will accept nutritional oils!

Recognize Your Arthritis by the Symptoms

The emphasis of this entire book is on oils and the battle to prevent dryness. Why wait for your joints to become worn and "frayed" at the edges from friction? You can prevent such a painful condition by starting now to obey the warning signals.

Symptoms of arthritis are the very proof in themselves that this disease is mainly a problem of dryness. Here is my list of danger signs.

SYMPTOMS OF ARTHRITIS

1. Dry, cracking, inflamed joints.
2. Dry skin, on various parts of the body.
   (Advanced cases show white, flaky skin over the ankles, knees or elbows.)
3. Dry scalp, dandruff in hair.
4. Dry, scaly ear canals, absence of ear wax.
5. Brittle or splitting fingernails, ridges in nails.
6. Wrinkles in skin, frequently at the sides of the neck.
7. Stretch marks in skin over muscles of arm and over the hips after substantial weight loss. This shows lack of elasticity in tissue. Proper dietary oils can even prevent stretch marks which follow pregnancy.
8. Loss of pigment in the hair (prematurely grey) earlier than is considered compatible with the person's age.
9. Itching in the area of the rectum.
10. Encrustations in the corner of the eyes.
11. Constantly "itchy" nose.
12. Buzzing in the ears.
13. Loss of color and complexion changes.
14. Stiffness upon arising.

15. Varicose veins.
16. Sterility.
17. Etch markings on teeth.
18. Bleeding gums.
19. Numbing and tingling in extremities.
20. Cold or clammy hands and legs.

If you have any of the above symptoms, perhaps you will readily agree that arthritis is a "drying out" process within your body. You may have one or many of these symptoms and still have arthritis. If any of these danger signs are present and they may come five to ten years before actual arthritis—it proves that you are susceptible to this disease. Take warning, now!

Important Experiments with Research Animals

To go on and prove even more conclusively that oils are the answer to arthritis, let's visit some laboratories and see the results of scientists working on "test animals." Doctors and research technicians have frequently done biological experiments with rats, for example, to determine the effect of oils. (Guinea pigs were found to be too sensitive to foods and environment, so rats were used instead.)

Medical experts set out to see what would happen to rats when all oil was removed from their diet. This experimental research of keeping rats on fat-free foods began way back in 1929. The early pio-

neers in this field were Dr. G. O. Burr and Dr.
M. M. Burr. In the *Journal of Biological Chemistry*
(Vol. 82, 1929, and Vol. 86, 1930) they reported the
following results.

RATS ON OIL-FREE DIETS

After 70 to 90 days on the diet, the rats had:
1. Dry, inflamed, swollen joints.
2. Dry and scaly skin: generalized throughout their bodies.
3. Inflamed, swollen, heavily scaled tail, with ridges.
4. Hind feet became red and swollen at times.
5. Dandruff in their hair on the back of their bodies.
6. Tendency to lose hair on the back, throat, and neck.
7. Sores often appeared on the skin, especially the face.
8. Blood in urine; kidney disease.
9. Female rats: irregular ovulation (longer cycles).
10. Male rats could not be induced to mate.
11. Retardation and gradual cessation of growth.
12. Consumption of water doubled.
13. 25% underweight.
14. Death due to kidney damage. (Usually found at autopsy)
15. Concretions in bladder. (Stone-like formations)
16. Shorter life span in general.

Do the above symptoms sound familiar? Yes,
many of them can be compared very closely with the
symptoms of arthritis in human beings. Oil deficiencies in the diet of the rats caused all these conditions, just as the lack of oils affects human arthritics.

Those experiments back in 1929 placed medical science on the right track. Since the rats were
allowed protein, minerals, oil-free vitamins, and
carbohydrates in their diet, it was felt that these
symptoms arose *only because certain oils were miss-*

EXPERIMENTS WITH RATS ON AN OIL-FREE DIET

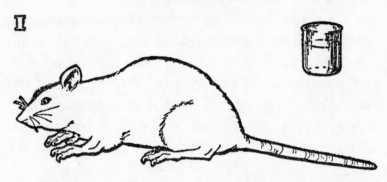

RAT NO. I fed on a diet containing oils. Normal water intake. Hair smooth and shiny, tail normal. Well-fed, healthy appearance.

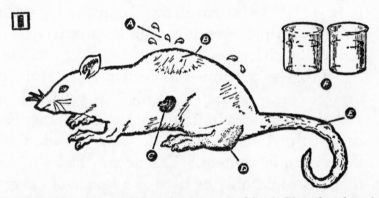

RAT NO. II. Oils removed from his diet resulted in: A. Water lost through diseased skin (not as urine). B. Hair contains dandruff and tends to fall out. C. Degenerative kidneys, urine bloody due to renal lesions which are immediate cause of death (in female rats ovulation becomes irregular and finally ceases). D. JOINTS BECOME SWOLLEN. E. Tail scaly and finally develops necrosis. F. Consumes twice as much water. (*Ref. Burr and Burr, Oser and Summerson, Practical Physiol. Chemistry.*)

ing from their food. The doctors named these missing factors "the essential oils."

In their efforts to cure the deficiencies in the
rats, the doctors used butter fat, corn oil, poppy
seed oil, supplemented egg yolk, linseed oil, lard,
cocoanut oil, and cod liver oil. Butter fat, for one,
could not do the job. This observation verified the
idea that the rats did not have a vitamin deficiency
disease. Because butter has oil soluble vitamins in
it.

Dr. C. E. Graham and Dr. W. H. Wendell
then reported in the *Proceedings of the Society for
Experimental Biology and Medicine* (Vol. 28,
1930–31) that while an oil could cure the dryness in
skin and scalp, it was limited in its effectiveness in
other oil deficiencies.

Progress continued under Dr. A. E. Holt. In
the *Journal of Pediatrics* (Vol. 6, 1935) Dr. Holt
and his associates admitted that until then they had
believed that all fats were the same. (Aside from
their vitamin content.) The doctors had also felt
that fats could only be used as a source of energy.
Now, in 1935, they had to take a different attitude
and re-examine nutritional oils. Dr. Holt discovered that infants on oil-free diets could develop
eczema and blemishes of the skin. The use of oil to
combat various ailments was now gaining in popularity.

Next, Dr. O. Turpeinen, in the *Journal of*

Nutrition (Vol. 15, 1938), wrote that he had tried some more experiments on rats to see how much of the *essential oils* were needed to prevent deficiencies. He found that very tiny quantities of oil would do the job—approximately <u>one per cent</u> of the diet. This now holds true for humans, too!

Then, from England came a vital observation. Four doctors, E. M. Hume, L. C. A. Nunn, I. Smedley-MacLean, and H. H. Smith, wrote in the *Biochemical Journal* (Vol. 32, 1938) that they objected to the irregular symptoms in the oil-free experiments which had been made. Not <u>all</u> the rats were getting kidney disease. The tails were not always corrugated. Why weren't they?

They soon discovered that when cod liver oil extract was given with the diet, kidney disease and other types of deficiencies did not appear. Here was cod liver oil coming into the picture as a recognized way to overcome oil deficiencies. These doctors were opening the door. This book will take you <u>through</u> the door to health. Chapter XVII is devoted entirely to cod liver oil and how it will aid arthritics.

Later, in 1941, two of the same doctors went even farther. In the *Biochemical Journal* (Vol. 35) Doctors I. Smedley-MacLean and L. C. A. Nunn wrote that in order to build new tissue in the body, substances like those found in cod liver oil were essential.

In addition to rats, arthritic research has had help from other animals, too. Dogs have been used in important experiments. The *Proceedings of the Society for Experimental Biology and Medicine* (Vol. 52, 1943) tell how Dr. A. E. Hansen and Dr. H. F. Wiese worked with canines. When subjected to oil-free diets, the dogs also developed dryness of the skin, dandruff in the hair, and eczema. Another observation about the dogs on the fat-free test was that they had lower amounts of blood iodine. When essential oils were replaced in the dog's diet, all these conditions disappeared.

Draw Your Own Comparisons

In this chapter we have watched outstanding doctors and scientists at work with experimental animals, and we have seen the tremendously damaging effect of oil deficiencies. Compare the symptoms which they created in test cases with your own signs of bodily dryness. The lesson for you is obvious. You need lubricating oils if you ever expect to rid yourself of arthritis.

We have traced the progress of modern research from 1929 to 1953 . . . by following the steps of leading medical men. Now, in the remainder of this book, we will show you how to use this accumulated knowledge for your own benefit.

Chapter IV

Combat Dryness in the Joint Linings and Cartilage

By now we have agreed that dryness is the major symptom of arthritis. We know, from the laboratory tests described in the last chapter, that this dryness often is general . . . it can appear in many parts of our body at the same time. So, where should we try to correct it first? What are the most important areas of the body which an arthritic should "oil" first?

Without question, you should rush lubricating oils to the linings of your joints and to the cartilage nearest your arthritic pains. These two parts—the joint linings and the cartilage—are the key points within your body. Lubricate them, and your arthritis will be gone. To show why this is true, let's discuss cartilage and linings in detail. You must learn all you can about these two features of your body, before you can fully understand your arthritis.

What Is Cartilage?

Present in every joint structure of your body,

near the ends of your bones, is an inert tissue known as "cartilage." It is a form of tissue, but it has no blood vessels, no nerves and no life. Cartilage serves as a pad or "cushion" near bones to prevent friction while the bones work and move at the joints.

Osteo arthritis, the most common type of all, is primarily an affliction of the cartilage. On this fact, more than 90% of all doctors agree. Tests have proven, time and time again, that osteo arthritis is cartilage destruction. This has been confirmed by X-rays, by autopsies, and through surgical pathology.

The question, now, is how can you nourish the cartilages and prevent their destruction. You cannot nourish them directly. (Only by osmosis, with iodized oil as we will describe in this chapter.)

Cartilage is made of mucin, albumin and sulfuric acid. During infancy, nature lays down cartilage cells which generate cartilage. Once formed, much like your second teeth, the cartilage does not regenerate with ease. This is so because it has no blood vessels, no nerves, and therefore cannot take direct nourishment.

By osmosis, however, iodized oil (like that found in cod liver oil) can reach the cartilage. This book maintains that oil is carried into the nearby joint cavity through joint linings which do have blood vessels. Through osmosis, the iodized oils filter into the cartilage and give the cartilage added elasticity. This elasticity keeps the cartilage from degenerating and wearing out.

Calcium Foods Are a Problem

In addition to keeping the cartilage elastic—by adding proper oils through correct diet—there is one other step which the arthritic should take. You should keep a close watch on how calcium enters your body. Be sure calcium bearing foods are eaten at the right time . . . and we will tell you the correct way to consume such foods later in this book.

Unless you are careful, calcium deposits may occur on your bones and complicate your arthritis. When not absorbed properly, calcium particles will attach themselves onto the bone near the cartilage. Spicules, daggers of calcium will knife into the cartilage and cause it to become frayed and worn.

As the frayed cartilage is subject to more and more mechanical wear, the cartilage finally disintegrates, adding to your acute pain and your arthritis.

While watching your intake of calcium foods, remember that their effect on your arthritis is only dangerous if they are eaten in the wrong way. If you set up a conflict between calcium foods and certain liquids, harmful deposits will result. Milk and calcium foods can be beneficial only if you know how and when to eat them. You will find additional chapters on this subject as you read on.

Doctors Examine Cartilage

The laboratory findings and facts about cartilage are by no means mine alone. For many years, scores of prominent doctors have been conducting extensive tests on cartilage. For example:

In 1920—

Dr. T. S. P. Strangeways wrote in the *Journal of the American Medical Association* that cartilage was able to take nourishment in some fashion. (Later, men of science agreed with his theory and said that cartilage is nourished by the process of osmosis.)

In 1934—

Dr. Ralph Pemberton of Pennsylvania reported that cartilage changes take place in osteo arthritis, and even in the later stages of rheumatoid arthritis.

In 1947—

Dr. Walter Bauer, a leading rheumatologist in Boston, described the progressive stages of cartilage degeneration which he and his associates found during autopsies. They reported that cartilage begins to deteriorate shortly after we become 20 years old.

Marie-Strümpell and Still's Disease

When you see a young man walking along the street with a "poker spine" (stiff and hunched), most often he has the Marie-Strümpell type of arthritis. (Named after Doctor Marie and Doctor Strümpell.)

Unfortunately, the victim must expect to walk in this frozen condition for the rest of his natural life. In his case, the cartilages between the vertebrae in his spine have become obliterated. They're gone, wasted completely away.

Even more pathetic is the children's type of arthritis known as "Still's disease." (Called by this name because Dr. G. F. Still of England first set forth its pattern.) In common with many forms of adult arthritis, Still's disease has wasting away of cartilage as a major symptom.

Correct Diet To Aid Your Cartilage

The doctors and medical experts mentioned above are only a few of the outstanding rheumatologists to whom we owe a vote of thanks. Hundreds of professional men like them also believe that research on cartilage will help solve the "wear and tear" phase of arthritis. This book maintains that we already have a way to aid the cartilage: Through proper diet.

To prevent loss of elasticity in cartilage—and to overcome dryness in the linings of the joints—certain dietary oils must be brought into our system with every meal. (The specific oils we need to do this lubricating job are named and discussed in later chapters of this book.)

We have just been reading a great deal about cartilage and how to keep it from "drying out." We have used cartilage as the main example because it particularly applies to people with osteo arthritis—and percentage-wise osteo arthritis encompasses the largest number of cases in America.

May we emphasize, however, that a similar "drying" process also occurs among victims of rheumatoid arthritis. In their case, all the dietary facts in this book still apply. If you have rheumatoid arthritis, the dryness starts in your joint linings instead of in the cartilage. Your "oiling" problem is therefore somewhat easier to solve. Why?

Because the inner structure of the joint lining does have blood vessels and lymphatic channels. Linings can take oil and nourishment directly, while the cartilage cannot. As long as your diet keeps the right nourishment coming in, the joint lining can send oils to the joint cavity. From there, some iodized oil will travel on even farther and reach your cartilage through osmosis.

So, as you can see, everything we have been discussing applies to rheumatoid arthritis, too.

Learn How Your Body Digests Food and Oils

Since much of this book will concern diets, food and eating habits, it might be wise for all of us to remember exactly how our digestive system works. Most of us had biology lessons in school, but we may be "rusty" or may have forgotten just what happens to a piece of food when we eat it.

To refresh our minds, let's trace the course of food from the moment we swallow it . . . how it is broken down by our digestive juices, and where it goes. . . .

First, we chew our food, masticate it in our mouth. Here, simple starches and sugars are acted upon by our salivary juices. Then the food enters our esophagus, the pipeline from the throat to the stomach. Immediately, the stomach begins digestive action. Foods are broken down into minute particles and mixed with the stomach juices.

Next, these particles are driven down toward the region of the small intestine. The digestive action on food in the stomach continues from three to five hours, until the food reaches a semi-liquid stage and the stomach becomes completely empty. <u>There is no digestive action whatsoever on oil or fat in the stomach.</u> The heat in the stomach merely changes the fat to oil.

At the end of the stomach, nature has provided

WHERE YOUR FOOD GOES

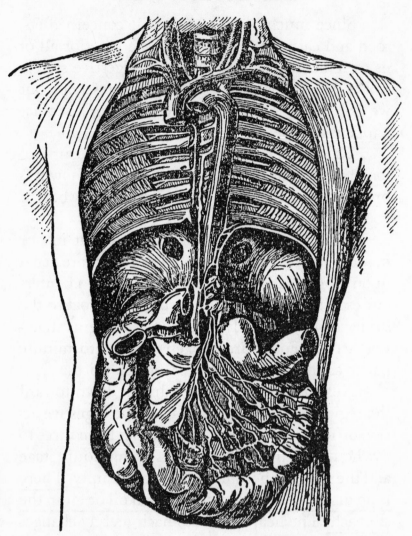

THE DIGESTIVE SYSTEM. . . . Trace the route of your foods and lubricating oils by following this drawing as you read this chapter.

a strainer-like valve which permits only semi-fluid materials to pass into the small intestine. This section of the small intestine is known as the duodenum. The passage of fatty or oily food substances through the duodenal region stimulates the action of the liver and the pancreas. The flow of bile and pancreatic juices begins.

Fat or oil which reaches the duodenum is emulsified by the bile salts. It is reduced to microscopic droplets. The useful food is now ready for absorption into the blood. (The non-useful residue is ready to be passed on through the large intestine and out of our bodies.)

Products like amino acids from protein, glucose from carbohydrates, minerals, and vitamins and oils are now transferred to some finger-like outlets in the walls of the small intestine. Everything except the oils must now go into the blood on the same route—they must pass through a pipeline known as the "portal vein." From the portal vein the foods go into the liver, for use by the body or for storage.

But let's go back and look at the oils, where we left them in the small intestine. When the oil droplets reached the finger-like outlets in the intestinal wall, they had their choice of two routes to enter our body. They can be collected by a trunk line known as the "lymphatic system" and shuttled around the liver, or they, too, can take the portal route.

Arthritics should get their oils to by-pass the liver . . . so the oils can continue on to the joints and do their lubricating job!

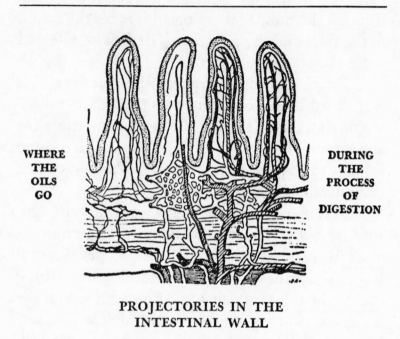

WHERE THE OILS GO

DURING THE PROCESS OF DIGESTION

**PROJECTORIES IN THE
INTESTINAL WALL**

Now, because of this chapter, we know why all arthritics need more oils—to save their cartilages and joint linings. Some readers might say: "I have been eating oil-bearing food for years—yet I still have arthritis. Why?" Because you have probably been making other dietary mistakes. As the next chapter will show. . . .

Chapter V

Faulty Diet Can Cause Arthritis

Arthritis is a disease of the body. A healthy body is usually indicative of a healthy diet. You are missing both.

Now, let us show you how to regain your most priceless possession—your health. By correcting your faulty diet!

Some people will say that food has nothing to do with arthritis. They'll claim that the disease is inherited. Such an idea is completely wrong, and here are some facts to show why.

Arthritis Is Not Inherited

This disease cannot be passed from generation to generation. What you do inherit are the dietary mistakes which your parents have practiced through the years. Faulty eating habits of your family make you susceptible to this dread disease.

You might say, "My husband and I have the same dietary habits. Yet, he does not have arthritis, and I do." Let us stop to analyze this puzzling fact.

Before you were married, very likely the diets of you and your spouse differed to some extent.

45

Today, your food choice might be the same. But, the order in which you eat your food probably differs. And the temperature at which you eat it. Temperature of food is a factor generally overlooked.

It is true that you both eat the same breakfast, but he likes butter on his toast. You both drink coffee. But you have sugar in yours, whereas he prefers his unsweetened and black. These minor changes often lead to major differences in your health.

In a hypothetical family, it might be that the mother will become crippled by arthritis, while her husband enjoys good health for another ten years. Then, gradually, he notices symptoms. The extra span of pain-free years for him could well be attributed to the habits mentioned in the previous paragraph.

Does a Change of Climate Help?

Let us turn to the children of our hypothetical family. Not so long ago, two of them—living in New York State—felt increasing pains in their hands. Now, in their thirties, they are starting to show the first signs of arthritis. Their older sister, who is forty-one, lives in California. Yet, she never writes of having any discomfort in her bodily joints.

Is it the climate which makes the difference? NO. Because as many Californians suffer with arthritis as do the inhabitants of any other state. Approximately 6% of the population in <u>every city</u> across the United States—be it East, West, North or South—is confronted with this common ailment.

Logically we cannot argue that the food in New York has less value than the food in Pennsylvania, Texas, or the Dakotas, for example. But Grandma and Grandpa in Ohio complain of their so-called "old age disease." And we have often heard them tell how their great grandparents in England were annoyed in later life by rheumatic conditions. That's why many of us think arthritis is inherited, because our parents or grandparents were victims.

You Are What You Eat

This book is <u>not</u> promoting health foods or its experts.

However, give Victor Lindlahr credit for a well-remembered statement, "You are what you eat." That is perfectly true.

If you are what you eat and you have arthritis, then for argument's sake, <u>you either ate something that caused your arthritis</u> . . . <u>or something you did not eat permitted its onset.</u>

We now have an approach to the cause of arthritis: Food or the lack of it. No one is saying that food in itself causes arthritis. We do maintain that one's food can lead to arthritis.

Based on thousands of laboratory tests, I conclude that arthritis is a particular kind of oil deficiency.

This deficiency of oil in the linings of your joints can be caused by many factors: Among the key causes are these:

1. Your food is oil deficient.
2. The oil in your food is the wrong kind. The joint lining will not accept valueless dietary oils.
3. The right oils are improperly digested. Most arthritics are victims of this faulty assimilation of oil-bearing foods.
4. The adrenal glands—a set of glands situated over the kidneys—are not secreting natural cortisone of "proper quality." This substance is vital to keep the oil in the joint lining.

Arthritis Complicated with Diabetes

If you are healthy and in the prime of life, most likely you pay little attention to selecting good foods from detrimental ones. You feel fine, because the body has to be pummeled a long time before you feel the effects of wrong foods. Then, suddenly you may find that you have diabetes or some other organic disease.

Some people can eat starchy foods for many years, until, as diabetics, they find themselves put on a low carbohydrate diet. It may take from a few days to many years for a faulty diet to cause an organ like the pancreas to degenerate.

Proper eating is more than just food. We must also know the order in which to consume food. Certainly we must start with the right edibles, good meat and vegetables, etc. But getting them properly digested and assimilated is another story. This book maintains—whether the problem is diabetes or arthritis—the order in which you eat your food is equally as important as the food selected!

Diabetes and arthritis frequently go hand in hand. The oil that an arthritic joint needs comes from the daily diet and is helped along by the digestive juices of the pancreas. But if we drink water, or even coffee with the meal, the duties of the pancreas are increased many fold. As a result, my findings show that this insulin-producing organ becomes dangerously overworked.

Arthritics . . . you are eating and drinking in the wrong order! You are nullifying the good effect of oil-bearing foods and you are placing an added strain on the pancreas.

In the chapters which follow we will present complete evidence to prove that arthritis is caused by a deficient diet. At all times, therefore, we must think of foods in terms of oil.

50

WHICH FOODS ARE BEST
FOR ARTHRITICS?

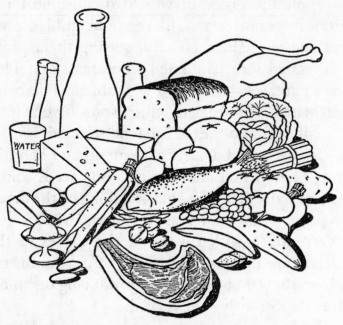

Some of these foods and beverages will help bring you relief from arthritis . . . others will hinder your recovery.

To learn the right foods from the wrong read the next three chapters . . .

Chapter VI

The Right Foods—To Help Gain Relief

Oil-bearing foods are everywhere. But the big question is what kind of oil do they contain. Several types of oily substances can be found in the same item of food. To gain relief from arthritis, we must seek a specific type of oil—found mainly in a limited number of fish and dairy products.

So, in this chapter, we shall name some of the most favorable foods for arthritics . . . explaining why and how they are valuable.

Milk Heads the List

Just about the perfect food is milk. It contains the right oil to serve dry arthritic joint linings. And milk has an all-important vitamin. Vitamin D. Without vitamin D in milk, this liquid would offer little compensation for those with rheumatic diseases.

A great many people with arthritis fail to drink milk, even though it is one of the best possible liquids to combat their problem.

When the arthritic drinks milk, he should take temperature into consideration. The temperatures of milk best suited to his condition are room temperature and lukewarm (up to 100° Fahrenheit). Do not favor hot milk, as it tends to constipation.

When you drink milk at room temperature, it can be taken anytime: before, with or after the meal. Even in between meals. As for cold milk, you can drink it safely before a meal—about five minutes before eating. Or, drink cool milk after a meal (but preferably not with the food, as it tends to congeal any other dietary oil).

Any amount of cold milk can be taken on an empty stomach. But, we repeat, to gain the maximum benefit from milk, it would be wiser to drink it at room temperature and at the end of the meal.

And remember, there are many kinds of milk:

1. Homogenized vitamin D milk
2. Buttermilk
3. Skimmed milk
4. Raw milk
5. Pasteurized milk
6 Powdered milk
7. Flavored milk
8. Goat's milk
9. Irradiated milk (exposed to ultra-violet ray)
10. Metabolized milk (cows fed irradiated yeast)

Each of the above types of milk yield different therapeutic results. But, skimmed milk and buttermilk produce a high tension on oil. They cause slower and improper assimilation of dietary oils, and if they are consumed with meals they have fattening powers.

Therefore, if an arthritic drinks skimmed milk or buttermilk, he should take it 15 to 30 minutes before the meal . . . or 2 to 3 hours afterward. These two kinds of milk offer the joint linings nothing. On the other hand, neither do they take anything from the body.

Most other milk (except powdered or flavored) can be enjoyed at any time. Before, with or immediately after eating. Of all types, we find that homogenized vitamin D milk offers the best asset to health. With pasteurized or raw milk, the cream separates out, taking with it much of the vital vitamin D and leaving about three-quarters of the bottle as skimmed milk . . . unless it is well shaken before using.

Multitudes of people offer excuses for not liking milk. It is fattening, they say, or it forms mucous. Women arthritics who fear putting on weight should still have some milk. It is that important. They do not need to take quite as much as others, however.

When cold, milk has a tendency to be more fattening than at room temperature. When taken at room temperature, it has additional value as a lubricating liquid. If obesity is your problem, simply cut down on the quantity.

One-half glass of homogenized vitamin D milk at the right room temperature is worth five glasses of cold milk—and in most instances will not put on weight.

Speaking of weight, one cup of black coffee with an oily meal has more fattening power than a glass of milk. The coffee turns against the oil in your food, and increases the energy potential of the meal.

Milk Is Not Acid or Gas-Forming

Many women who have kept away from milk for years may find, when they start drinking it again, that it forms mucous or that it causes flatulence (gas).

Even these people, so distressed, should not give up milk. They should take smaller quantities, and not with every course. At the start, six ounces of milk, at the correct temperature once a day, is enough. Gradually, over a period of months, they should train their bodies to accept a six or eight ounce glass at every meal. The mucous condition, gassy feeling or any milk allergies can be overcome with patience.

Goat's milk, years ago, had the reputation of being helpful in alleviating arthritic pain. There is some basis of fact for this idea. Goat's milk is more highly-emulsified than ordinary cow's milk and therefore this would indicate better assimilation.

Let's remember, however, that homogenized vitamin D milk is not the complete answer to arthritis. We are not advocating a diet solely of milk. Many other correct foods are needed, too . . . in order to provide sufficient quantities of the oil soluble vitamin.

Milk Is Not Calcium Forming

Often we hear that people are afraid to drink milk because it is calcium forming. This need not happen. Over 100,000,000 Americans drink milk every day. And these straight milk drinkers do not develop bumps of calcium on their bones. It is when you start mixing milk or cream in coffee, tea, cocoa, etc. that this trouble originates.

The explanation is simple. Pasteurized milk is subjected to high temperatures. This heat causes the oil in milk to envelop the calcium particles. When you put milk in coffee, you create a new tension on the calcium. This seals the calcium even tighter so that it is not assimilated so easily. As a result, calcium deposits are left in the wrong tissues or on the ends of bones, such as on fingers.

If you drink a glass of water after a glass of milk (or even after a dish of ice cream) it is little wonder that the calcium does not go into bones, nails and teeth. You do not give the calcium an opportunity to be utilized normally. Never think you are getting your milk when you add it to coffee. Coffee is essentially water, and is not compatible with milk.

Why Adulterate Your Milk?

Adding flavoring to milk—such as chocolate, strawberry, coffee or malt—is sweetening the perfect liquid. It only promotes obesity and does not lubricate the linings of your joints. When the arthritic alters milk, even by adding ice cream, he is tampering with one of nature's best foods. Remember, most adulterated milk is basically skimmed milk.

Whole milk is 87% water and has very low tension on the oil in a meal. But skimmed milk and buttermilk have very high tension on oil. Drinking skimmed milk with a meal sounds less fattening to the average person, but because of its tensive quality, it turns other dietary oils into fat.

Any arthritic drinking skimmed milk with the meal is increasing the waistline, while the poor old joint linings remain dry.

On the other hand, whole milk—with its low tension on the oil in the rest of your meal—allows more of the correct oils to go on to serve in a lubricating capacity.

Summed up, the best milk for arthritics is homogenized vitamin D milk.

Oil from Butter

Butter is a reasonably good weapon in the fight against arthritis. But do not overdo it. Especially if you have a tendency to be overweight. Butter does not contain enough vitamin D to justify having a person indulge in it excessively.

Like milk, butter contains the oil soluble vitamins, A and D. The A vitamin is good for the linings of the eyes and skin, while the D vitamin benefits the linings of the joints. I repeat, if there is a tendency to put on weight, cut butter to a minimum. Milk is far more important.

The best way for a victim of arthritis to use butter is on whole wheat toast. Or on hot cereals or hot vegetables. If you place butter on cereal, you will nullify and cancel the essential vitamins if you add sugar, honey or molasses. Sugar cheapens oils. When butter is used on wheat cakes, why kill off the good effect of the butter by adding syrup!

Oatmeal would be an excellent choice of cereal on which to use butter. For sweetening, however, if you must have it, use saccharin or a sugar substitute. Not raw, white, brown or any other kind of true sugar.

Salt, we have found, should be kept low in the diet. But one eats so little butter, it makes no appreciable difference whether he selects the sweet or salted variety.

In choosing between butter and oleomargarine, take butter in every instance. Because of its iodine value. Butter does not ravage the body for iodine, whereas oleomargarine has this tendency. Butter, according to our tests and experiments, gives the skin lustre. While in the case of oleomargarine, the skin may become greasy with the wrong oils. Margarine may have the same food values, but butter does not usurp iodized oil.

Today, many women try to save pennies by using vegetable oils for cooking and baking. In families where there are arthritics, this habit should be minimized.

Arthritics definitely should limit themselves when eating cookies, cakes, pies and starches made with any kind of oil. Sweets defeat our purpose. Sugar cheapens the value of the best lubricating oils.

Butter makes a baked potato taste delicious, but eat the mineral-laden jacket, too. Although potato is starchy—it is of "superior" starch-quality. Cake, pie, candy, sweets and refined foods are of the "cheap-inferior" starch-quality and "ravage" tissues of the body.

Potatoes, whole grain breads and cereals are approved. If you tend to obesity, keep even approved starch-like foods to a minimum.

Egg Yolk Has the Right Oil

Eggs are enjoyed by most people every day. It will be helpful for arthritics to know that the value of eggs is not affected by the color of the shells. The most important part of the egg is the yolk. And it doesn't matter whether the yolk is light or medium yellow.

Farmers everywhere realize that the color of the yolk is determined by the chicken's environment. Many farmers confine their flocks to keep the yolks a true yellow. Roaming chickens, it seems, yield darker yolks. Actually, the color is not important, but the vitamin assay is.

If you let your imagination create ways to prepare eggs, you could compile an almost endless list. For arthritics, however, the best methods of preparing eggs are these:

1. Three-minute boiled eggs
2. Poached eggs
3. Coddled eggs
4. Raw egg nog (no sugar)

To gain the maximum vitamin D from an egg, serve a three-minute boiled egg on whole wheat toast. Scrambling an egg—or combining it in other forms of cooking—is throwing away many benefits. As for a hard-boiled egg, the only advantage it offers is that it is harder to digest.

If, as we grow older, we are unfortunate enough to develop heart or gallbladder trouble, we are told to restrict our consumption of eggs. Children eat eggs every day and never suffer any ill effects. Yet, adults who do the some thing often get into health difficulties. Why?

The explanation is not due to just "growing older." The damage is caused by the difference in the dietary habits of the two age groups. Children generally follow their eggs with milk, a liquid with low tension on oil. Adults, on the other hand, drink coffee, a high tension liquid. Since coffee and eggs do not mix well, a life-long habit of using the two together causes trouble later in life.

Let's not forget that coffee is essentially water. When taken with coffee, egg yolk then turns into a rubbery material which taxes the gallbladder and heart. Respect the egg yolk. It can offer health, or, when not used wisely, can be a detriment.

Oil from Chickens

Chicken broth is traditionally a favorite food. Whether you like the broth or not, chicken soup is a remarkable liquid and it has been used for generations among the sick.

Yes, we recommend chicken broth for arthritics. It has the right type of oils and vitamins.

When eating a drumstick of a chicken, have

you ever taken time to notice the gristle and the lining adjacent to the joint? Next time, look closely. If the gristly cartilage is a golden yellow, the chicken's diet has been substantially good. When the yellow or colorless gristle (cartilage) is not present at all, that chicken has had arthritis!

Chickens Have Arthritis, Too

Whether fowl, capon, roaster, fryer or broiler, barnyard creatures can eat their way into arthritis. The farmer can tell when a chicken has joint ailments. He looks at the fowl, and can see their legs swell and the way they limp. We may well wonder why chickens get this disease. Is their diet wrong?

For the most part, chickens eat corn or mash. Corn contains traces of vitamin D in its oil. The oil is there, but like human beings, chickens do not always properly assimilate what is in their food.

Like people, chickens make the mistake of drinking water with their meals—thus disqualifying the essential vitamins. The chicken (or person) who tries to mix oil and water violates one of the oldest rules of chemistry.

When chickens drink water with their corn or mash, the dietary oil turns from lubricating oils into surplus fat. Excess deposits of oil are then found under the skin, or wherever tissue will store it. The result: an arthritic chicken.

When it comes time for you to cook a chicken, watch out for these faulty deposits of fat in the bird. They will not serve your arthritic body, they'll just fatten you.

Trim away any chicken fat under the skin or in the body cavity of the fowl. If you do not remove this fat before making soup, then skim it off the soup dish.

The only oil worth consuming from the chicken is found in the normal gristled drumstick. There is not enough of vitamin D in a single drumstick with a healthy lining to be of really major help. But the healthiest chicken broth is made from these drumsticks and the giblets. It is just as easy to make chicken broth from a pound of drumsticks as it is to cook the whole chicken.

If you take time to serve chicken broth, do NOT be tempted to serve it in the following forms:

1. Chicken soup with rice
2. Chicken soup with noodles
3. Chicken soup with dumplings

Remember, rice, noodles and dumplings make the soup starchy . . . the wrong kind of starch. And arthritics must abstain from such carbohydrates if they want to become well and stay well. Brown rice or whole grains are superior to the polished variety, and they may be added in small quantities if you feel that you must have something in your soup.

Again, let us examine the case of a farmer with his chickens—to draw some interesting comparisons for human arthritics. On progressive farms today, many ranchers take steps to give their flocks of chickens a balanced diet. In addition to corn and mash, the fowl are provided with carotene (supplemented carrot oil). Also, they receive some kind of fish liver oil, combined with their food. This helps the chickens to further productivity and prevents rickets.

With humans, we know that liver oil from the codfish is used successfully to help prevent rickets in children. Fish liver oil and carotene contain vitamins A and D—and often also have the fertility promoting vitamin E.

The A, D and E vitamins mentioned, in their natural state, exist as oil soluble vitamins. Each vitamin has a job to do and a specific place to go. Vitamin A, as we know, is valuable to the eyes and their linings. Vitamin D, as used against rickets, is of great aid to the minerals for bone and joint formation.

Vitamin E is recommended for fertility. It is found in supplemented carotene. So, when a chicken gets its sustaining food with supplemental vitaminized oil for a few months, there is a very noticeable difference in its appearance. The joints grow straight, with no swelling. The feathers have lustre, the skin is elastic and normal. The eyes are good and the nails of their feet are firm. All this, because oil has been added to the diet!

Oil Vitamins in Fish

Fish, too, have oil which can prove helpful to lubricate the dry linings of an arthritic person.

Not enough fish is eaten by the American people. We are known as a nation of meat-eaters. But it is fish, not meat, which contain more of the oil soluble vitamins.

Ask those who eat fish why they do so. You'll receive a variety of answers:

1. They like fish
2. It is inexpensive
3. Their husbands go fishing. Someone has to eat it
4. Because fish is "brain" food
5. Because it is Friday

Whatever your reason for being a sea food fan, remember that there are all kinds of fish. . . . Some better for us than others. Not every fish has the vitamins-in-oil which are best suited for arthritics.

If you have arthritis, you may choose either salt or fresh water fish. Broiled fish has all the advantages over other styles of preparation. Why cook your fish . . . you'll lose the vitamins. Broil it.

When choosing fish, make your selection from

those types which contain the most vitamins A or D. Recommended as the very best are:

1. Mackerel
2. Halibut steaks
3. Salmon steaks
4. Sardines

If you don't like to eat the skin of the fish, you are losing many health essentials this food has to offer.

When you don't consume the skin, you can make up for some of the loss by eating the dark brown meat near the skin. It is in the brownish meat that goodly quantities of fish iodine are trapped. Iodized oil is very beneficial to arthritics. It is the right kind of oil. I'll have more to say about this important oil in a later chapter of this book.

A SIGN OF FAULTY DIET
And a possible symptom of future arthritis

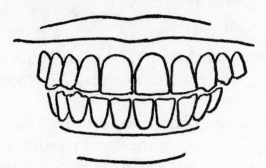

NORMAL TEETH
(above)

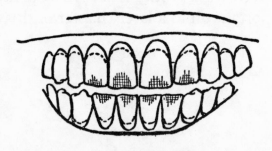

ETCHING OF ENAMEL . . . and . . . RECESSION OF GUMS

Examine your teeth. Etch marks, erosion or gums starting to recede can mean the presence of arthritis—or that the disease may soon come and make you an arthritic.

Chapter VII

Fruits and Their Effect on Bodily Oils

When you eat a lobster dinner, or southern fried chicken with your hands, a restaurant often serves you a finger-bowl. Next time you receive the little dish of water take particular notice of the tiny piece of lemon that came along, too.

Did you ever stop to think <u>why</u> that slice of lemon was served to you? Because, as you wash your hands, the lemon is supposed to <u>cut away the oils</u> from your soiled fingers. Lemon does undermine oils, and arthritics should never forget this fact.

Why do beauticians use lemon juice rinses on women's hair? To wash away excessive oils from the scalp. From observation and medical reports, we now know that this violent cutting action of lemons also takes place inside a human body.

If an arthritic turns to lemon juice in an attempt to cure his affliction, he is ignoring the lessons taught by the practices described above.

The Lemon Juice Myth

As a last resort, many arthritics will seek an overnight cure by drinking excessive amounts of lemon juice. It seems that centuries ago lemon juice was found to be beneficial for scurvy. Simultaneously, it supposedly aided a number of persons with arthritic symptoms. The idea flourished and it was carried on as a rumor for nearly three hundred years.

Starting in the 16th Century, people tried to cure scurvy by taking about two teaspoons of lime juice once a week. This was added to some solid part of the diet. When lime juice was not available, a fresh vegetable—like turnip or some greens—was tried as a substitute.

After this lime legend became widespread, it was suddenly changed to lemon juice. Instead of two teaspoonfuls a week, it grew to taking a glass of lemon juice per day. Then, four or five glasses of lemon juice were advocated—and not to fight scurvy but to "cure" arthritis. It didn't work, not for arthritics certainly.

Speaking of scurvy, the ancient Romans believed that parsley alleviated the disease. The Dutch became convinced that sauerkraut would help them. The Moors also tried to overcome scurvy with lemon juice. The herb doctors in England attempted to cure it with watercress. North American Indians used a tea made from pine needles with "magic success."

Hundreds of years have passed since scurvy was reported in the 16th Century. Now, as recently as August 10, 1951, the Rochester (N.Y.) *Democrat and Chronicle* reported scurvy cropping up in Tallahassee, Florida—in the heart of the citrus industry.

In Florida, people who had all the citrus juices they wanted—growing in their own backyards—found themselves with the marks of scurvy. They had loosening of teeth, loss of appetite, pain in the arms and legs.

Is this the penalty for drinking citrus juice, rather than eating the fruit in moderation? Does this mean that if your gums bleed, they will bleed even more from too much citric juice? Ironically enough, the answer to both questions is yes. And I'll explain why in more detail as you read on. . . .

The myth which led to the use of lemon juice for arthritis has gained in popularity. Today, many crippled and maimed arthritics use it in frightening quantities, all to no avail. To those who think this juice does help, look at the way your skin and body are drying out. Evaluate the damage you have done yourself. Look at the color of your hair. Is it becoming grey prematurely?

Lemons Are Not the Answer

Time has now borne out conclusively that lemons are NOT a cure for arthritis. Instead of being helped, many arthritics become worse and some become permanently disfigured. Fruit sugar in any citric juice—particularly lemon juice—has a parasitic affinity for joint and skin linings and pigment. In the case of the joint lining, it may well hasten degeneration and its resulting deformity.

If lemons were the answer, there would not be millions of arthritis sufferers in all parts of the United States. There are lemons for sale in nearly every neighborhood store in the country—and still the number of arthritics grows larger and larger.

Next, someone discovered that lemon juice in water would help relieve constipation. No doubt this is so. It is said that lemon juice clears the blood. Perhaps it does—but at a terrible price. Let this be a warning to you if you are tempted by lemons. Observe and gauge joint pain daily. Watch your skin, nails, scalp and hair as they become drier and drier.

Why jeopardize your arthritic body—to rid yourself of constipation by means of lemon and water—when constipation can be conquered in so many other less harmful ways?

In 1947 the reputable Mayo Clinic in Rochester, Minnesota, issued a warning about water and lemon used for constipation, colds and rheumatism. Clinically they found that it erodes the enamel of teeth, a very hard substance.

If lemon mixed with water has this awful power against tough tooth enamel, think of the effect of this citric juice in undiluted form! It would be proportionally more disastrous to the body internally.

Medically, we know the acid of the juice is reduced to alkali . . . but in reduction, what price does our poor body pay? The urine, pretty well stabilized at an acid level throughout life, can be alkalized by drinking copious amounts of lemon juice. What a terrifying effect it must have on the bloodstream and its oils? Summed up, lemon juice kills off the lubricating oils we need most—prevents their proper digestion and circulation to our joints!

For arthritics a little lemon juice sprinkled occasionally on a salad or used as a flavoring on fish is condoned. But that is where the use of lemon juice should stop.

Under no circumstances should people with arthritic tendencies indulge in lemonade during hot summer months. If an arthritic is seeking early and lasting health, eating lemons or drinking lemon juice should be forgotten indefinitely.

Limes

Closely associated with the lemon is another fruit, the lime. Most people do not consider actually eating limes. They should not. Arthritis sufferers should even refrain from drinking lime rickeys or any drink containing that particular juice, because of its drying effect on the bodily oils.

Grapefruit

There is still another citric fruit which finds its way into the diet of many arthritics. They have been led to believe that it is rich in vitamin C—and it is. We refer to the grapefruit. It, too, has a severe drying effect on the oil being distributed throughout your body.

When sugar is added to grapefruit, even more disastrous damage is wrought. Note your joint pains as they get worse, your skin as it gets drier. Five years after an arthritic becomes well, grapefruit can be eaten occasionally without too harmful results.

Until then, while the body is trying to correct oil deficiency, grapefruit and grapefruit juice should be omitted. There are many, many fruits— rich in vitamin C—which do not tend to dry out oils. For example, do eat, enjoy and benefit from apples, peaches and pears.

There have been many diets offered by accepted authorities as beneficial to arthritics. Very often you will see citric fruits have been eliminated because of the acid properties. Many other dieticians agree with me on this point.

People with arthritic tendencies have often discovered the "citric truth" by themselves. Sufferers have sometimes recognized the stinging pain which followed their excessive intake of citric fruit. But these victims of arthritis too often ignored the pain signals. Their complaining became known as the "acid myth."

I repeat, go easy on the use of grapefruit and lemon juice!

Now, let's go on to discuss the most popular citrus fruit of all. . . .

Oranges

A popular breakfast is a quick one . . . which a person can gulp down. In their haste some mornings too many arthritics will just drink a glass of orange juice and call it a meal. Unfortunately, when you drink orange juice—hastily or otherwise —it has a drying effect on the skin and joints.

But . . . EATING AN ORANGE IS SOMETHING ELSE AGAIN, it is not so detrimental to arthritics. When you eat an orange, the saliva in your mouth alkalizes it. Keep from drinking plain orange juice, because its fruit sugar and citric acid are in a combination which attacks bodily oils.

The orange is only 1% acidic. The lemon and grapefruit are 7%, with 7 times the drying effect.

The longer a person has had arthritis, the more he should abstain from plain orange juice. One year after being fully relieved of pain, the arthritic may eat sections of an orange in a fruit salad. Or, an occasional whole orange, well masticated.

*EVEN FOR PEOPLE NOT THREAT-
ENED BY ARTHRITIS, HEALTH AUTHOR-
ITIES RECOMMENDED THAT CONSUMP-
TION OF ORANGES BE LIMITED TO TWO
OR THREE PER WEEK. AS YET, SCIEN-
TISTS DO NOT KNOW HOW MUCH AC-
TUAL VITAMIN C OUR BODY REQUIRES.*
Concentrated frozen citric juices should be
omitted altogether from the arthritic's diet.

*What Doctors, Dentists, Medical and Health Magazines
Are Saying About Citric Fruit . . .*

Experimental work is now being done on citric fruit, and doctors are using live rats in these
tests. Let's examine some of the results of their
experiments. The following paragraphs will give
you a condensed version of what the medical profession reports in recent years about citric fruits.
Dr. C. M. McCay of Cornell University, as
reported in *The Journal of Nutrition* (Nov. 10,
1949), made a study on four groups of rats. He
sought to discover the approximate rate of destruction on teeth, caused by various beverages. The
doctor used tomato juice, orange juice, cola beverages, and distilled water. Distilled water had no
effect on the teeth. Tomato juice etched the enamel
slightly. Orange juice caused a marked erosion on
the teeth in only six months' time. (The effect of

cola beverages will be discussed in the next chapter.)

In his book *Diet in Sinus Infections and Colds,* Dr. E. V. Ullmann reasoned it was unnecessary to drink huge amounts of orange and grapefruit juice to get our quota of vitamin C. He suggested, on the contrary, that minute amounts be consumed.

The *Journal of the American Medical Association* (Feb. 3, 1951) announced that apple, grape, pineapple, orange and grapefruit juices crack the enamel on teeth.

From France, in 1947, Professor T. Bondouy of the School of Medicine in Tours pointed out that an excess of fruit juices in our diets could cause impaired digestion—generally a forerunner of stomach ulcers. He also described experiments wherein the vapors or essence of lemon and orange killed several strains of microbes—including the deadly diphtheria and typhoid germs. He announced further that grapefruit, lemon and orange juices produce intestinal gas and abdominal flatulence.

Doctors J. Yeagley and D. Cayer set out to test "the general belief that fruit juices are 'acid' and that they aggravate the symptoms of peptic ulcers." By November of 1948—as recorded in the *North Carolina Medical Journal* of that month—they had proved that orange juice could bring pain and burning sensations.

From the Proceedings of the Staff Meetings of the Mayo Clinic, Rochester, Minnesota (March 5, 1947) came a report by two dentists. Doctors E. C. Stafne and S. A. Lovestedt found that in a study of 50 patients using lemon juice for one reason or another, every one of them was suffering from varying degrees of erosion in his teeth because of the ascorbic acid of the lemon. They discouraged anyone from drinking lemon juice daily. They also found that after lemon had been used too long, mere brushing started wearing away the borders of the teeth.

In July of 1950, Dr. H. Hicks presented interesting reports on his patients in the *Journal of the American Dental Association*. Some of them complained of sensitivity in the mastication of apple skins and celery. His patients reported hives, mobile teeth, bleeding gums, buzzing in the ears, dizziness, constant headaches, constant tiredness, enamel around fillings washing away, and foul breath.

When Dr. Hicks eliminated their orange, lemon and grapefruit drinking—and let them eat moderate amounts of raw fruit—their complaints practically disappeared. In place of vitamin C from citric juice, Dr. Hicks substituted cabbage, green peppers, and other vegetables rich in C. He went so far as to conclude that ingestion of excessive amounts of citrus fruit caused deleterious effects on the whole system, as well as on the teeth.

Reporting in the August 1951 issue of the same journal, Dr. C. D. Miller in Hawaii found that pineapple, grapefruit, guava, and java plum juices had more demonstrable erosive effect on the teeth of rats—worse effects than eating the same fruits.

At the *Biochemical Research Foundation*, St. Petersburg, Florida, Melvin E. Page, D.D.S., stated that fruit juices put undue strain on the mechanism of the body.

J. I. Rodale, editor of *Prevention*, a magazine devoted to the conservation of health, wrote that excessive citric juices could be very harmful to the body. He added that this discovery about citric juices was the most unusual health fact he had come across in a lifetime of research.

Anyone seeking a more complete listing of the effects of excessive fruit juices on the body will find 33 most interesting pages on this subject in *Prevention* magazine of October 1951.

Fruits in General

Raw fruits, like apples, bananas, apricots, cherries, peaches and pears, offer minerals—and they are needed by the body for good health. Apples, eaten as nature grew them, are beneficial to everyone. But, if you bake them, you gain little.

Apple juice and pineapple juice are oil cutting, and arthritics should abstain from these juices. "An apple a day" is a time-honored proverb . . . but do not drink, bake or cook it.

(With baked and cooked apples there is the chance—as with cooked vegetables—of destroying the vitamins in your food.) You may certainly eat all the apples you desire.

Drinking pineapple juice should be curbed. But arthritics may eat pineapple slices now and then without too much harm. As for the pear, because of the sugar content even in the raw fruit, it is best that you limit your consumption of pears.

If you enjoy prunes, they may be had raw or stewed. Chew them well. Do not drink prune juice; its sugar goes after oil.

Bananas have only fat producing oils. If you don't have too much excess poundage, now . . . if you're not worried about your waistline . . . go ahead and enjoy bananas. They won't affect your arthritis.

In this chapter we have discussed fruits and juices. Now, let's go on to examine other beverages. . . .

Chapter VIII

Modern Beverages—A Help or Hindrance?

Whatever else our 20th Century may become famous for, history will remember that this was the age when "soda-pop" was born—in a big way! Our American capacity to invent new "soft drinks" is endless. I'll have quite a bit to say, in this chapter, about "pop" and "fizz water" . . . a menace to arthritics.

But, first, let's consider the most common beverage of all. . . .

Coffee

If you have arthritis, you may still drink coffee without harmful effects. But only if you drink it at the right time in relation to your meals.

Coffee will not conflict with the oil in your foods, if you drink the coffee at least ten to thirty minutes before a meal . . . or at least three to four hours after a meal. Black coffee is more advisable. Do not add white sugar to any coffee, but substitutes like saccharin may be used.

Tea

We have inherited from England the habit of tea drinking. For the sake of arthritics, I wish we hadn't. The tea habit is most drying to the oils of the joint and skin linings. Tea is bad for arthritics, because of its tannic acid content. Adulteration with sugar, lemon and ice also makes tea a dangerous liquid for arthritics—when used excessively.

If you know how to drink coffee, 100 cups of coffee do not disturb your bodily oils as much as one cup of tea. If you have a painful shoulder or knee and you were to spend a few weeks consuming tea, you would undoubtedly be able to feel added pain in your sensitive joints.

A Doctor's Opinion on Tea

Dr. T. Short's well-known book, *Discourses on Tea*, points out that people with neuritis and other rheumatic diseases, shortness of breath, liver disturbances—and those who are sallow and anemic—should refrain from drinking too much tea.

Carbonated Beverages

Now, how about carbonated beverages? "Soda pop" seems to be practically replacing milk in the American diet. To show you how bad this is, let's make a simple test. . . .

Take a good oil, like butter, and add it to a glass of carbonated soda pop. See for yourself how the butter becomes obliterated. It is immediately reduced to harmful oil, full of gas and sugar.

Carbonated soda is an oil parasite. Soda literally eats and destroys oil and its value. Arthritics

should abstain completely and forever from carbonated beverages, if they want to become well and
stay well.

Soda pop, seltzer water, fizz water, sugar water,
tonic—whatever you call them it's still a carbonated beverage. If you doubt the destruction of oil,
drop a few ounces of most any carbonated cola
drink on the hood of your automobile. Notice what
happens to the oils in the car paint! You'll shudder,
if you imagine the same terrible action in your
body.

Epidemics of disease often occur in the summer—when the drinking of carbonated beverages
is at its peak. Why do the number of cases of appendicitis and poliomyelitis increase in hot weather?
Added drinking of soda may be a contributing factor.

Can gas and sugar in carbonated soda pop devour the oil and fat in the fatty covering of the
appendix? Leaving the appendix exposed to inflammation? (This is what happens in the case of
joint linings, and perhaps it could apply to the appendix too.)

It also follows that carbonated beverages can
undermine the sheath of oil which covers nerve
tissues. Nerve cells would be exposed, permitting
the nerves to be hosts to an infiltrating virus like
that of polio.

Recently, there have been several articles published suggesting this very same idea about polio. Yes, polio virus would find it very difficult to attack an oil covered nerve. Strip away the oil, and you invite danger.

Look at the inroads polio is making into older age groups. Is the higher intake of carbonated water a possible explanation?

What Doctors, Dentists, Medical and Health Magazines Say About Carbonated Beverages

In the *Annals of Western Medicine and Surgery* (February, 1952) Dr. G. Blumer reminds us that the *Journal of the American Medical Association* has been calling attention to possible harm caused by the chronic use of soft drinks. Some soft drinks contain harmful drugs; most of them cause deleterious chemical reaction to the body. And, too often, soft drinks are substituted for more healthy items of the diet.

Dr. Blumer also indicates his desire to see parents educated about the possible dangers in the excessive use of soft drinks. He suggests that a law be passed requiring that ingredients of soft drinks be indicated on their labels. He urges that there be more search and investigation on the effects of carbonated beverages.

Dr. C. McCay of Cornell University fed his set of experimental rats many types of fruit and cola beverages. The lemons, grapefruit and oranges were highly erosive on the enamel of teeth. But the cola beverages were far worse!

Remember, many soft drinks contain phosphoric acid.

In his experiments Dr. McCay with his collaborator, Lois Hill, suspended human teeth in cola solution. They found that the calcium of the teeth would dissolve in the phosphoric acid in just two weeks' time!

In the *Journal of the American Dietetic Association* (April, 1952) Dr. C. D. Miller reported giving carbonated drinks to 129 rats along with their food. His conclusions: Flavored sodas, colas and all carbonated beverages erode the enamel of the teeth.

The *Pennsylvania Medical Journal* (May, 1944) has a warning for us, too—in Dr. H. H. Turner. He stated the belief that the alarming increase of Americans forced to wear eyeglasses is the result of the carbonated beverage habit. Particularly because the young children of today drink so much soda pop.

An instructor in Clinical Nutrition, Dr. M. J. Walsh (University of California) has prepared charts demonstrating that soft drinks have no value as food.

Doctors E. C. Stafne and S. A. Lovestedt of the Mayo Clinic's Dental Division have reported that human teeth exposed to cola drinks and acid beverages show faster process of decay. These beverages would lead to greater mechanical wear, through brushing the teeth and chewing.

The work of Dr. C. McCay aroused the interest of *Consumers' Report*. In July, 1950, they published findings on 13 common soft drinks. *Consumers' Report* evaluated the drinks for their acid content. The following table shows the result of the tests:

	Brands	Acidity (pH)	
Colas	6	2.4	
Ginger Ale	12	2.7	
Lime, Lemon & Lime	7	2.9	The lower the number
Cherry	7	3.1	in the column on the
Raspberry	4	3.1	right, the greater the
Orange	11	3.2	acid content.
Root beer	4	3.4	
Grape	6	3.6	
Cream soda	11	3.9	7 is neutral, and is ap-
Sarsaparilla	15	4.0	plied to water.
Cocoa cream	3	4.3	
Club soda	10	4.7	

Generally, the lower the acidity, the more erosive the acid beverage is on tooth enamel.

Another reason why carbonated soda pop is so harmful is that a large amount of the gas is assimilated by the body, because there is no atmospheric pressure in the stomach.

J. I. Rodale, editor of *Prevention* magazine wrote in a 1952 issue that citric, tartaric or phosphoric acid were frequently used for flavoring carbonated beverages.

We know, from excessive users of citrus fruits,

that citric and tartaric acids are injurious to the body. Editor Rodale was particularly concerned about the youth of America and their tremendous consumption of soft drinks.

Millions of youngsters are drying out their systems. They are destroying the proper assimilation of bodily oils. Acids fight oils. It is little wonder that more and more American young people are becoming victims of arthritis.

So, in closing this chapter on carbonated beverages, one fact is evident. Many medical authorities agree . . . arthritics should stay away from soft drinks. As you have read, the evidence is all against these liquids.

We have discussed "soft" beverages . . . but what about the "hard" kind? Cocktails? Liquor? The next chapter, rather logically, will cover drinking. How does alcohol affect arthritics? Read on, for information and more helpful findings. . . .

DAILY HABITS AFFECT ARTHRITIS

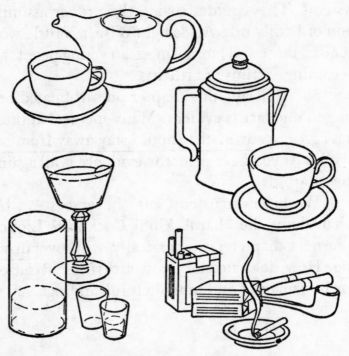

DRINKING TEA, COFFEE, LIQUOR . . . SMOKING . . .

Will all of these habits do any real harm to an arthritic? Or can we enjoy these pleasures and still gain better health?

FOR THE ANSWER . . . SEE THE NEXT CHAPTER . . .

Chapter IX

About Our Habits . . . Eating, Drinking, Smoking

Every night is not New Year's Eve. And with the exception of a few celebrations throughout the year, most of us are probably just "social drinkers." When it comes to liquor, you don't need this book to tell you that drinking of the "lost weekend" type is injurious to anyone's body. But the question is . . . how does a normal amount of liquor affect arthritics?

Alcohol may be enjoyed if you drink it at the proper time, before meals. Do you take your drinks straight or mixed? If you mix them, do you mix with water, carbonated water, club soda, sweet cream, or just ice cubes? It makes a great difference to your joint linings and your arthritis. Take your liquor straight or with plain water, not the carbonated kind.

When you over-indulge with hard liquor and do not eat correctly for many years, the nutritional deficiency and the liquor can lead to a scarred liver. Worse, if you mix your drinks with carbonated products, you may eventually scar your joint linings as well.

The order in which you drink liquor is all important. Even an occasional highball or cocktail should be taken at least 10 to 30 minutes before you eat. Never with the meal. In other words, keep liquor away from your dietary oils while they are being digested.

Beer is a form of carbonated beverage, so drink it sparingly. Whenever you do drink beer, again, make it before mealtime. Or at least three hours after eating.

Smoking

When anyone starts discussing the subject of drinking, the next topic of conversation is usually "smoking."

You may have the habit of lighting a cigarette while eating. You may wonder if you are also lighting the way to arthritis. My research does not indicate that smoking can ever do anything to dry up the oil in your body. We have found, however, reports that excessive smoking can cause arteries to contract. Such contraction could lead to joint tissue damage. The whole problem probably hinges on whether or not you are a chain smoker.

Go ahead, enjoy smoking. Just use moderation.

What is moderate smoking? Well, you should certainly draw the line after one package of cigarettes each day. Use this as a comparable yardstick in regard to cigars and pipe-smoking.

Eating Habits

There are several minor practices which occur during our meals and have a direct bearing on arthritis. Seasoning our food, for example. Should we use vinegar, mayonnaise, special oil dressings on salads, etc.?

Vinegar must be condemned. It is not compatible with the oils we are trying to digest. For the same reason, the use of French dressing should be minimized at all times. Even though there is a small amount of vinegar in mayonnaise what we want to avoid is vinegar used in its liquid form. Therefore moderate use of mayonnaise or 1000 Island dressing (or some emulsified types of salad dressing) is not objectionable.

Sugar Undermines Your Diet

White sugar, added to liquids, is particularly injurious to the arthritic. An over-abundance of sugar throughout your life causes the walls of your intestines to degenerate. Then, the sugar particles travel to the joint linings and burn up the oils.

Sugar destroys the very oils we are trying to save. For example, when we withdraw joint fluid and measure the sugar content in a <u>normal person,</u> there is approximately 80 milligrams per 100 centimeters of fluid. In an arthritic, with a fasting stomach, the percentage of sugar would be about the same. But . . . give the arthritic with a degenerating intestinal wall one bottle of carbonated soda pop and in twenty minutes the sugar content of the joint fluid will <u>triple!</u>

Oil is burned or cheapened by "inferior-type" carbohydrates (sugar). Avoid sugar in liquid form, granulated or as honey or molasses.

We have been commenting on various habits which play a part in causing arthritis. In the next chapter we will consider one of the most common fads of all. The practice of running to so-called health charts every time we need an answer to a dietary problem. Do these charts serve any real purpose? You'll find the answer, starting on the next page.

Chapter X

Do Charts on Health Have Any Value?

Since the days we went to grammar school, we have been shown colorful charts listing the number of calories, proteins and vitamins in hundreds of different foods.

Remember the sign near the blackboard showing a glass of milk, a loaf of bread and a nice red beefsteak? Next to each picture were a lot of figures which we could add up to give us the total carbohydrates and minerals contained in what we ate. We were taught, from school days on through our adult life, that these charts were our best guide to health. Now is a good time to ask: "Have we been misled?"

My belief is that such charts are helpful. But . . . they are also missing two of the most important facts of dieting. Two facts which can cause the entire chart to be meaningless and misleading.

No chart ever says anything about the correct temperature of foods. And they never list any order in which to eat the items.

Have the experts who draw these charts forgotten that the value of each food will change due to temperature and position in the meal?

To prove the seriousness of this charge, let's

91

go back and take another look at that schoolroom
chart which starts off showing a glass of milk. . . .

Milk has vitamins, protein, carbohydrates, etc.
But what the chart does not show is that if you drink
milk cold, it has a different effect than when you
drink it warm. There is no mention of the fact that
if you drink milk at room temperature it will be digested more completely—and your body will receive more of the vitamins, protein and carbohydrates. Just changing the temperature can change
the whole count and totals on those so-called "perfect" charts.

Feed a new-born infant on cold milk, instead
of lukewarm milk, and you will have sad proof by
checking the condition of the baby's skin, scalp and
nails. Both types of milk will nourish, but the
warmer kind will do a tremendously better job.

Nowhere on the magic charts do they tell you
whether to drink your glass of milk before your
meal, while eating, or afterward. Again, the vitamin and calorie count, etc., will be changed. This
change in food value can occur because the value
of the milk will depend on how thoroughly it is
digested and assimilated. It will depend on whether
the milk runs into conflict with other foods which
you are eating at the same time.

What Health Charts Say About Fruit

Every decent health chart always recommends

fruit. Oranges, grapefruit, pineapple, etc., all are needed to give the body vitamins and minerals. We agree. But why don't the charts show the difference between the methods of consuming fruit? The value sworn to on the charts is changed when you switch from eating raw fruit to drinking it in juice form. The point we are making is that charts are incomplete in their information.

Charts neglect to take any notice of what ailments a person may be suffering from. You may have some special physical condition which will alter the totals published on charts.

A pregnant woman, for example, may need more fruits than are normally listed for the average person. (Incidentally, obstetricians highly recommend juices for expectant mothers.) My research indicates, however, that sharp fruit juices withdraw oils of all types from the skin. Juices contribute to the loss of elasticity of the skin, and lead to the appearance of stretch marks. Therefore, we recommend that during pregnancy—in fact, for all people, always—fruits should be eaten, not poured in.

Charts on Eggs Leave Much Unsaid

Eggs are considered an ideal breakfast food and appear on every nutrition chart. This is fine, we recommend them for arthritis too. Unless an allergy prevails or you have a gallbladder ailment, arthritics should enjoy eggs frequently.

But here's another case where the charts fell short. Why didn't they print something about the method of cooking eggs. The nutritional value of eggs is drastically altered by the way they are prepared. For instance, when you scramble eggs you make it impossible for your digestive tract to assimilate the egg yolk properly. Arthritics should rely on boiled three-minute eggs.

MEATS are pictured in brilliant, appetizing colors on every "Vitamin Chart." Yet, you are never told by the diagrams that over-cooking will destroy the very vitamins you are seeking. Arthritics, especially, should beware of tossing out the vitamins in the cooking water. Instead, broil your meats, medium rare.

VEGETABLES should be treated with the same care. Avoid excessive cooking. Use a pressure cooker, or serve vegetables raw, when possible.

WATER is the most neglected item of all when the health chart experts do their art work. We never see a picture of a glass of water along with the colorful foods. Diluting your foods, while they are being digested, can raise havoc with the figures on the chart. Drinking water can reduce the value of vitamins, protein, minerals, etc. Arthritics should realize this threat, and you can read more about it in Chapter XII.

Most of the foods which health charts list do contain water soluble vitamins, as well as oil-

soluble vitamins. These substances are very important to our bodies. The oil types of vitamins are vitamins A, D, and E. If the oils and fats carrying these
vitamins into your body suddenly have their chemical structures changed—because you are simultaneously drinking water—how can these vitamins
serve as true vitamins for body maintenance? They
have been diluted or practically destroyed.

Examine Yourself, Then Your Diet

Before you use charts, diagrams or special
menus, it would be a good idea to determine
whether you actually need to change your eating
habits. Are you really suffering from any dietary
deficiency?

It is simple enough to recognize whether or
not your body is being nourished by a balanced
diet. These are some warning symptoms:

1. Color is missing from your cheeks (Protein
   deficiency or poor protein assimilation)
2. More and more cavities occur in your teeth
   (Carbohydrate imbalance)
3. Bones break easily, if you fall (Mineral deficiency)
4. Night blindness, or need for stronger eye
   glasses (Vitamin deficiency)

Naturally, there are many more symptoms of

diet deficiencies. We have mentioned but a few. However, there are many good books on such subjects available in the library. This book will now return to the subject of arthritis.

Because too many arthritics are over-impressed by "health charts," we have been trying to point out in this chapter the most obvious shortcomings of such listings.

Again, we maintain that temperature and the order of eating foods are far more important than just "calorie counting."

Chapter XI

Shift the Liquids in Your Diet

If health charts cannot be relied upon—as we saw in the last chapter—what are the rules which can guide an arthritic to health? One basic instruction takes precedent over all others. Shift the liquids in your diet, or lose the value of your entire meal!

The relationship of foods and liquids, and how to realign them at mealtime so they will not conflict within your body will be the subject of this chapter. In many ways, what you are about to read now is the most important part of this whole book.

To make it clear and simple, we will start by considering foods. Then, we will go on to liquids, and we will recommend actual breakfasts, lunches and dinners.

There are only five types of food. That is, all foods contain at least one of the following five benefits:

1. Protein
2. Minerals
3. Carbohydrates
4. Fats (Oils)
5. Vitamins

97

Rarely is anyone in America short of proteins. We are the world's largest meat consumers, meat packed with protein. Minerals are readily available in any raw vegetable or fruit. Carbohydrates are found in plentiful amounts in bread, cereals, etc. Fats (oils) abound in butter, eggs and milk. Vitamins can be had from fish, fowl and green vegetables.

Suppose, for a test case, we look at a typical family. Suppose they are eating all five classes of food, in the proper proportions. Yet some members of the family are well, and others are ill. Why? Because each of them drink different liquids, at different temperatures, at different times, during and between meals.

Their choice can include milk, tea, coffee, water, beer, or dozens of other liquids. Each of these liquids has a different tension on oils in their food. It is this tension on oils which decides how useful the oil will be to the body. High tension on oils will force your system to use more digestive juices to break down your food. Which means more wear and tear on your organs, particularly the pancreas and gallbladder.

To show you this process of digestion at work —so you can see the damage which liquids can do— let's take a typical day of eating and follow the route of your foods. The day starts with breakfast . . . here are "good" and "bad" menus. . . .

Typical Breakfast (Not Recommended for Arthritics)

> Chilled grapefruit juice
> Scrambled eggs and bacon
> Bread and butter
> Coffee with cream

Breakfast (Suitable for Arthritics)

Eat your food in the following order:

> Buttered whole wheat toast
> Soft boiled eggs
> Glass of milk (room temperature or
> warm) (Approximately 400 calories)

First, look at the breakfast marked NOT RECOMMENDED FOR ARTHRITICS. It reads like a normal menu for the average person. What's wrong with it, then?

The foremost error is starting the meal with grapefruit juice. The arthritic is immediately pouring into his empty stomach a bath of astringent juice. He is cutting into oils, and drying out his system. Next, he eats the bacon and eggs with bread and butter. The pouch-like stomach now has 6 to 10 ounces of grapefruit juice joined by scrambled egg and some fatty bacon. Scrambling the egg means its egg yolk will never be assimilated as oil but as energy. Bacon offers the wrong kind of oil to overcome arthritis.

Cold bread with butter needs more digestive juices to split the oils. Instead, the arthritic should have had warm toast with melted butter.

Lastly, comes the coffee. When the water in coffee gets to oils, like those in butter and eggs, it increases their fattening potential. What we're looking for is a lubricating potential. A small beaker of cream or milk is added, along with two teaspoons of sugar. Butter and coffee are not compatible. Sugar burns up fat, deteriorates the oils.

If dry cereals are substituted for bacon and eggs, the cereal is usually drowned with cold milk. The temperature of the cold milk will congeal oils, not aid them. As you can see from the above paragraphs, during this simple breakfast the arthritic has made at least seven major mistakes. So, now, let's examine the right way. . . .

The Approved Breakfast for Arthritics

On the menu marked SUITABLE FOR ARTHRITICS the first difference you will note is the absence of fruit juices. Drinking fruit juice will devour, delay, or change the power of oils. Your bread is listed as the whole wheat variety, and toasted. Chew it well. The butter on the toast will start the oil flowing.

When eggs are served, it is wise to soft boil them. When substituting cereal for eggs, select a good one like oatmeal. We want to avoid refined and excessively starchy cereal. In any event, do not use sugar on cereals. If cereal is eaten at breakfast, be sure that the milk you pour on it is of room temperature.

Do you feel that you must have more vitamin C? Then try a more concentrated supplement of vitamin C, use bottled tablets of ascorbic acid. This commercial preparation may be added to any portion of the breakfast. Or, liquid vitamin C in oil form can be bought in any drugstore, and used at breakfast time. This is even better.

End your morning meal with lukewarm or room temperature milk, not water. This will keep the flow of oil mounting and rolling into your body. If you drink coffee in place of milk, drink it black and shift it to the beginning of the meal.

LUNCHEON can be a waste of time, if you don't understand the correct positioning of foods. That is, you will be gaining no ground in your fight against arthritis, if you eat a meal like this. . . .

Typical Lunch (*Not Recommended for Arthritics*)

Ham sandwich
Glass of water
Pie or cake
Tea or coffee

Lunch (*Suitable for Arthritics*)

Eat your food in the following order:

Grilled cheese sandwich
Tossed salad (no oil, no vinegar)
Glass of milk (room temperature or
warm) (Approximately 600–900 calories)

Most likely, before the average person begins
the ham sandwich in the NOT RECOMMENDED
LUNCH, he has a harmless appearing glass of water. He's wrong, right at the start, if he drank it
three or four minutes before eating. It takes your
stomach closer to 10 minutes to release the water
into your system. Otherwise it will just be waiting
there in your stomach to dilute the value of your
foods.

The ham sandwich may prove of little use, too. Most ham has fat either on its border or interspersed throughout the meat. When digested, ham fat yields no vitamins. It has worthless oil for arthritics. Instead of being improved with butter, the ham is often spread with mustard.

Perhaps the sandwich was started first, and the victim drank water to wash it down. Or his tea was too hot, so he added more water. In either case, the oil-line to the joints is still waiting for oil. And the water is still breaking down, damaging, or slowing up the process of oil-delivery.

Before he finishes the tea or coffee, he starts eating the apple pie. Raw apple is good for you, but baked apple in pie crust is only adding starches to your system—cheapening whatever oil is present. The more starches, the harder it is to recover from arthritis.

Adding cream or milk to iced coffee or tea has two harmful effects. It results in poor digestion of dietary oil. It also forces the gallbladder to resplit the cheap oils coming from the ham and the dessert. No wonder your bloodstream cannot deliver the necessary oils. And you are inviting a gallbladder condition.

Comments on the Approved Luncheon

The RECOMMENDED LUNCH, on the other hand, helps answer your oil deficiency problem. With this diet we begin by eating an "oil food." It can be a grilled cheese sandwich on whole grain bread. Or, a slice of buttered toast. Or even a soup or broth of some kind.

Green lettuce, green celery, cucumber, and carrot make an easily digestible and nutritious salad. It will provide important minerals and vitamins. If you wish, skip the toast, soup or the grilled cheese sandwich, and drink half of your milk. Then eat your salad. Finish the meal with the remainder of the milk.

Lunch must never contain fruit or vegetable juices, carbonated water or highly rich desserts.

DINNER can be either the best or the worst meal of the day for arthritics. The menu below is a comedy of errors, due to improper positioning of the food. . . .

Typical Dinner (Not Recommended for Arthritics)

Cocktail, beer or wine
Shrimp entree
Iced water
Small tenderloin steak
Vegetables
Ice cream
Coffee

Dinner *(Suitable for Arthritics)*

Eat your food in the following order:

Cup of soup or broth
Broiled steak, medium rare
Two vegetables, one raw
Apple
Glass of milk (room temperature or warm) (Approximately 800-1200 calories)

The meal NOT RECOMMENDED begins with a beverage. Either the hard or soft kind. Either is a mistake, taken too close to the start of a meal. But sometimes the place where you are eating or your social surroundings force you into a peculiar corner regarding your diet.

Suppose you are eating dinner at some smart hotel or restaurant. You may have to keep in fashion by having a cocktail, beer or some wine to start. Any liquor mixed with club soda or carbonated ginger ale is tremendously drying to oils in your body. If you must have liquor to be polite, ask that it be served straight or mixed with plain water. Beer, and liquor in moderation, is approved—providing you drink it at least 10 minutes before your meal.

Next, you enjoy your shrimp cocktail. For arthritics, nothing gained, nothing lost.

By this time, the waiter is back again to show off the fine service of the restaurant. He refills your goblet with ice water. As you wait for the steak course, you pass the time by sipping. If there was any oil at all in the shrimp cocktail or its sauce, the oil now doesn't have a chance. It is congealed, frozen, and has to be re-emulsified. What's more, you have filled your stomach with water which can now just lay in wait to drown the value of your coming steak course.

All the vegetables and other foods still to be eaten in your meal will suffer because you are drinking water.

The Approved Dinner, and Why

The RECOMMENDED DINNER begins with oil-bearing soup or broth. You can then enjoy your steak, but pay attention to how it was prepared. Broiled steak is best for arthritics. Broiled medium rare, from a lean cut of meat. In this manner your body will receive all the vitamins and proteins.

Raw fruit (like apples or peaches) can be eaten for dessert. Chew them well and reap their harvest of minerals and vitamins. Use fruit in season, but not the citric variety. (See fruit list, p. 150.)

In essence, this chapter has endeavored to show how many oil-free liquids can destroy the balance in a so-called "balanced diet." By shifting "conflicting" liquids to their proper place in each meal, you can double your chances to recover from arthritis.

Just beware of detrimental liquids, particularly excessive quantities of water. The correct use of water by arthritics is so important, we are publishing a whole chapter on this vital subject. The next chapter. . . .

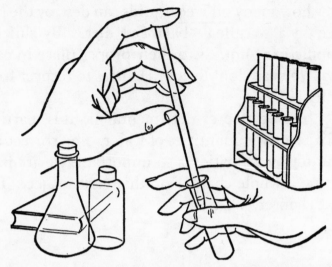

My hundreds of laboratory experiments with ordinary drinking water proved the effect of water on the human system.
ARTHRITIS has been found in the bones of prehistoric
monsters, in alligators and in human skeletons. The cause can
be improper habits while drinking water.

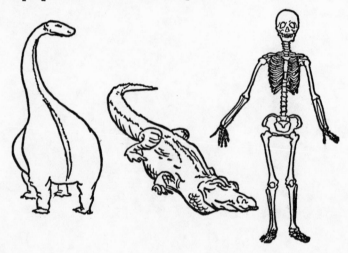

Chapter XII

Drinking Water—a Curse or a Blessing?

Arthritis and drinking water are definitely related. They have been down through the ages. To understand the role which water plays in your arthritic condition, we must go back through history.

If we study the effects of water on animals, we can learn a great deal and draw comparisons with our own bodies. Which animal should we use as a "guinea pig" for our tests on arthritis? A chicken, a monkey, or a rat? No, let's use a dinosaur.

Arthritis appeared in animals thousands of years ago, even before man was on the earth. In fact, the earliest cases of arthritis probably developed about two hundred million years ago! The victim's name was not Jones or Smith. It was Tyrannosaurus Rex, or some such dinosaur-like title.

Yes, paleontologists have found symptoms of arthritis in the vertebrae of prehistoric land monsters. Examination of fossils show that the backbone of these creatures closely resembles the spinal arthritic changes of modern mankind. In the museum of the University of Kansas, one can examine the remains of an arthritic sea reptile, dead more than 100,000,000 years. This prehistoric swimming beast was known as a mosasaurus. Its fossils plainly exhibit chronic arthritis in the backbone and other joints.

A Really Old Case of Arthritis

In other museums there are numerous fossils proving the susceptibility to arthritis in ancient men and animals. Chronic osteo arthritis predominated then. Arthritis has been found in the small triassic and the diplodocus dinosaurs, as well as in the oreodon, a mammal. The primitive ungulates of 50 million years ago also had it.

The crocodile of 15 million years ago, the camel of 1,800,000 years ago, the cave bear and the sabre-toothed tiger of 500 thousand years ago—all show the markings of arthritis.

Arthritis Strikes the Earliest Man

Of the early two-footed animals known as "man," skeletons show that the Ape Man had a deformed spine. The "Java Man" was afflicted with bony spicules of the long bones, typical of osteo arthritis. The "Lansing Man," along about the year 500,000 B.C., had multiple arthritic involvement of the lumbar vertebrae, first metatarsal bone, and the hip and knee joints. The Neolithics, the Ptolemaic Egyptians (who inhabited Alexandria during the Greek and Roman periods), the Copts of early Christian times, and the pre-Columbian Indians of America—all have borne the curse of arthritis in their bones and joints.

The symptoms in these mammalian, reptilian, and amphibian fossils do not vary much. All these cases definitely belong in the category of osteo arthritis. They all could be diagnosed as "wear and tear" on the joints. Yet, not every dinosaur and not every man had the disease. Some managed to stay well. Which means there must have been other causes—in addition to "wear and tear"—that led to their arthritis.

Was "Old Age" Responsible?

What, then, did prehistoric animals and men have in common with the osteo arthritics of today? The process of aging has been suggested as the probable cause of their ailments. But the fossils of some "young" dinosaurs show arthritis, too. Just as the disease often strikes humans today in their thirties or forties. Age must be ruled out as the answer.

The chronic arthritic of today is invariably troubled with constipation. It is a little late to check for this symptom in prehistoric mammals. All that is left of them are some bones and teeth. By the same token, it is too late to study the changes in skin, scalp, nails, etc., of ancient Egyptians, Greeks, and

Romans. We will never know whether they lacked lustre, sheen, natural oils, or showed other signs of dryness.

No records were ever kept to show whether early-day arthritics had kidney or thyroid difficulties. Perhaps their muscle or liver tissue showed degeneration. Muscle and liver tissue specimens are now being examined in some arthritic clinics. These tests are comparatively new, and are not widely used as yet. We hope they will be soon.

As in the case of modern human beings, climate was <u>not</u> the basic cause of the arthritis in prehistoric animals. The beasts were found living all over the world, in all climes, and they still had arthritis.

Certainly, we cannot accuse prehistoric animals of drinking carbonated soda pop, seltzer, tea, or other acid beverages. But they did have one liquid in common with us. Whether it was 200 million years ago, or last Friday night, arthritics drank <u>water</u>.

Water, Water Everywhere

Mosasauruses swam in water, as did the Egyptian crocodile. They drank a lot of it, too, during their meals, while munching on live fish. The Ape, Java, and Lansing men all were known to quench their thirst with water. They had no diet controls and no knowledge on how to shift their liquids to the proper part of their meal. Can this be the key to the cause of arthritis down through the ages?

Do not get the impression that water alone can cause arthritis. Not in the sense that one glass of water can create pain just because you drink it with your meal. But it does slow down digestion, lead to faulty assimilation of food by-products, and cut off the supply of oil to your joints.

How Much Water in the Human System?

Let's remember that we all have a great deal of water in our bodies already. The average man has approximately 100 pounds of water in his chemical makeup. This liquid forms about 70% of the body. Blood is 90% water, and our human bones are 22% water. This liquid—H_2O (two parts of hydrogen and one part of oxygen)—is an essential part of every cell in our body.

Men can survive longer without food than without water. If you lose just 20% of the body's water supply, it can mean dehydration and death.

We should take note of the fact that there are several different kinds of water. Distilled water, spring water and the regular reservoir type, for example. Water can be hard or soft. Hardness depends on the presence of mineral salts like sulphur, iron, and magnesium. When an arthritic thinks that mineral water is helping him keep regular, it is probably due only to the vast quantities he is drinking at regular intervals, rather than to the mineral content.

How Water Serves Us

There is no doubt that water is vital to our health, if we drink it at the proper time. It aids in digestion, assimilation, circulation, and excretion. Through water, body heat is distributed quickly and in the right proportions. When too much heat is produced, the body cools itself by an air-conditioning method of its own, using the lungs and skin.

Water also helps transport waste products from tissues to the blood, and then through the kidneys. It serves as a watery cushion for our central nervous system. All embryos develop in a water environment. It is said that even our backbones shift continuously in a watery medium.

Sometimes an arthritic in a hospital depends on water for physical treatments. If he's in a wheelchair, he may need water therapy. It could be whirlpool baths, or exercises in a warm pool. Buoyed up, he is able to flex and work his muscles.

Water Habits Cause the Damage

We repeat, water itself is beneficial. The wreckage it causes in our bodies comes from the method of drinking it. When water is consumed in our meals and how.

Bad drinking habits, unfortunately are often passed on to us by our parents. If, as children, we see a pitcher of water on the table at mealtime, we naturally continue this habit through our adult years. This practice can lead to arthritis, and we later wonder if we inherited the disease. No. We inherited the water fad.

Take a test family of four children, all girls. They grow up, get married, and scatter to their new homes in different parts of the country. They take with them their water habits. If their husbands were not accustomed to seeing water on the dinner table, the men will now be introduced to the water craze.

In the average American home the lady of the house may drink water with breakfast. Her husband does not, but he likes vichy water for luncheon, at the restaurant near his office. Their young son drinks water for lunch, instead of milk. Their teenage daughter drinks a glass of water every night before going to bed. She has heard that it is good for the complexion. The whole family is wrong. And they are flirting with arthritis, paving the way to become victims of this dread disease.

How Much Water Do We Need Daily?

Science tells us our bodies require a cubic centimeter of water for every calorie which our foods produce. Therefore, if you eat a 2,100 calorie diet each day, you need approximately 2,100 cubic centimeters of water. This amount, put into the usual receptacle, is equal to eight glasses of water!

No one would be foolish enough to recommend that you "Drown" yourself by drinking eight glasses of water every day. Besides, there is no need to, because other foods contain great quantities of water.

Milk, for example, is 87% water. Coffee has even a higher percentage. So arthritics will drink less water, we have prepared a special chart. The figures and foods below will prove to you that you are receiving plenty of water at every meal. Read this helpful list, and use it as a guide:

Foods	Percentage of water
Egg	74
Cottage cheese	74
Cream cheese	53.3
Cheddar cheese	39
Butter	15.5
Veal	71
Liver	70.9
Chicken	67.1
Round steak	67
Lamb	66
Chuck roast	65
Frankfurts	64.3
Corned beef	57
Ham	53
Spareribs	53
Pork	50
Oysters	87.1
Codfish	82.6
Salmon	67.4
Tuna	57.7
Sardines	47

Cucumbers	96.1
Squash	95
Lettuce	94.8
Tomatoes	94.1
Celery	93.7
Radishes	93.6
Asparagus	93
Spinach	92.7
Cabbage	92.4
Cauliflower	91.7
Broccoli	89.7
Carrots	88.2
Onions	87.5
Potatoes	77.8
Green peas	74.3
Cantaloupe	94
Watermelon	92.1
Oranges	87.2
Peaches	86.9
Apples	84.1
Pears	82.7
Bananas	74.8
Rye bread	37.6
Cake	26.8
Cornflakes	9.3
Oatmeal	8.3
Walnuts	3.3
Peanut butter	1.7
Yeast, bakers	70.9
Yeast, brewers	7
Wheat germ	11

The above listing offers conclusive proof that water can reach our bodies in adequate amounts while we eat. There is never a need to drink eight glasses of water a day on top of all these water-bearing foods. Three glasses—taken well before meals —should be plenty.

Millions of Americans who are now living

healthy, normal lives, drink as little as one glass of water daily. They do not become dehydrated, or suffer any ill effects. Remember, too, that saliva, stomach juices, bile, pancreatic, and intestinal juices all have the necessary water to break down your food by natural means. This is accomplished without help from an extra glass of water.

Your body often decides for itself how much water it really needs each day. When it has enough, your system passes off excess liquids. Approximately four and one-half pints of water are eliminated every 24 hours. Most of it in the form of urine. Water is also released in your exhaled breath. Or, as perspiration through your skin surfaces.

Ten Best Suggestions To Be Water-Wise

The wisdom of using proper water habits has been shown throughout this chapter. By now, arthritics should be ready to accept some helpful recommendations. Your recovery from arthritis might depend on how well you follow a correct water regime.

For easy reference, and to summarize the leading requirements, here is a basic set of ten reminders:

1. Drink your water at least 10 minutes before your meal.
2. After meals, wait at least 3 hours before drinking water.
3. No water with your meals.
4. Water is good for you upon arising, but try to drink it

warm, one hour before breakfast. Taken that early, the water is mildly laxative.

5. Never drink lemonade, or water flavored with fruit.
6. Never add water to milk.
7. Avoid using aerated water, flavored carbonated water or seltzer types.
8. Hard water, soft water, fluoridated water, chlorinated water, spring water, distilled water—it makes little difference to your arthritis. The TIME of intake is important.
9. Never add water to soup. (For instance, to cool it off once it is cooked and served.)
10. When you drink coffee (which is water) be sure it is at least 10 minutes before or 3 hours after your meal.

Remember the above laws on drinking "oil-free" liquids, and you will have taken a major step toward relieving your arthritic pains. You will be protecting the oils in your body, rather than "washing them away."

What these pages have been trying to say is that many liquids have high surface tension on oils. TENSION is the key word. Tension caused by water prevents your foods from being digested properly. When you create high tension inside your body, it repels digestive enzymes and disrupts the flow of lubricating oils.

Water has the highest surface tension of any food on earth. Therefore, it could be your greatest enemy. Depriving your arthritic joints of those very essential oils!

PROOF . . . RESULTS OF LABORATORY TESTS

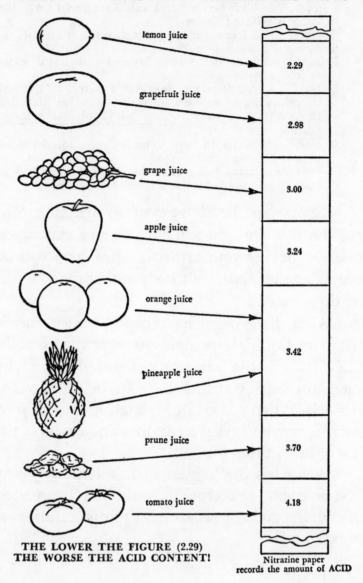

lemon juice — 2.29

grapefruit juice — 2.98

grape juice — 3.00

apple juice — 3.24

orange juice — 3.42

pineapple juice — 3.42

prune juice — 3.70

tomato juice — 4.18

**THE LOWER THE FIGURE (2.29)
THE WORSE THE ACID CONTENT!**

Nitrazine paper
records the amount of ACID

Chapter XIII

Acids in Food Lead to Sensitivity

Next to water (when you drink it at the wrong times), the most dangerous element in our food is acid. Most everything we eat has some form of acid in it. Unless we carefully watch our "acid intake" at every meal, we can become victims of "gassy stomachs," ulcers, nausea or many other bad reactions by our sensitive bodies.

Therefore, now that we have examined foods to learn their water content (in the last chapter) it is equally important to learn the "acid content." If water can harm lubricating oils needed by every arthritic, imagine how much more damage acids can do to those oils!

Before we show how acids in foods actually injure the sensitive bodies of an arthritic, let's see how scientists measure acidity. How they determine whether acid is present in our diet.

In scientific laboratories, doctors and research technicians frequently use two types of specially treated paper to make their tests. Material known as litmus and nitrazine paper is used. When a strip of blue litmus is placed in any liquid containing acid, the litmus paper turns red. If the liquid is non-acid, the blue litmus keeps its blue color.

It has been found, for example, that approximately 10,000,000 quarts of water yield one gram of hydrogen ion "acid." The degree of acidity depends upon the number of hydrogen ions in the solution. In mathematics, the logarithm of 10,000,000 is seven. For the purposes of simplicity, then, water is referred to as having a pH of 7. This figure "7" is the basis for measuring acids in foods. Anything above 7 is alkaline, anything below 7 is acid.

After litmus paper has shown there is some acid present, then the scientist uses nitrazine paper to measure how much acid is there and how strong or caustic it is. Nitrazine paper in the presence of water does not turn color, but remains a dusty greenish color with a value of seven. Acid content in foods and liquids decline from 7 down through 4.0, and lower.

Milk, when tested in this way, turns out to be slightly acid. It has a pH of 6.6. If milk were 7, it would have no acid at all. Therefore, we can see how very small the acidity of milk really is. That's one reason why we recommend milk for arthritics, because of its extremely low acid content.

To keep acids away from lubricating oils should be the main goal for anyone who has arthritis. No wonder we condemn fruit juices. Look at this chart and recall what you have learned about the number 7. Remember, the lower the pH, the more acid in the food.

THE HIGH ACID CONTENT OF FRUIT JUICES

FOOD	pH LEVEL
Lemon juice	2.29
Grapefruit juice	2.98
Grape juice	3.00
Apple juice	3.24
Orange juice	3.42
Pineapple juice	3.42
Prune juice	3.70
Tomato juice	4.18

The above list speaks for itself . . . a plain warning to arthritics.

Most of the above foods have also been found to etch teeth in experimental animals, and humans.

If they can erode tough tooth enamel, no wonder these juices cause reactions in more sensitive organs of your body. Many arthritics give up juices voluntarily, when pains in their joints increase. We maintain that the pain results from oils being dried out by citric, phosphoric, or tannic acid.

The Experience of Leading Doctors

Medical men know, and you should realize, that sugar is an acid, too.

Dr. R. Pemberton has established that arthritics suffer from a delayed sugar removal tendency. When arthritics are given sugar solutions on an empty stomach, the sugar content in the lubricating oils increases sharply. Again, acids (sugar) are deteriorating the oils in your joints. Dr. C. McCay of Cornell found in his research that the saliva of men averaged a pH of 4.4. Women have a surprisingly lower average of 3.8. These acid values were constant throughout the day.

Teeth are considered subject to erosion when the pH in the mouth is brought below 3.5. After that figure, the salivary juices cannot cope with anything more acidic. Arthritics are risking even their teeth, when they drink juices and liquids which are below pH 3.5.

Above we have shown how women have more salivary acid (3.8) than men. This may be one big reason why there are more female arthritics than male. (The disease strikes three women for every man.) Why? It could be because women have more acid in their saliva to start with, and thus cannot accept added quantities of acid in their foods. Their bodies cannot neutralize food acids as readily as men.

The Acid Content of Your Blood

We have been discussing the acid content of saliva and other fluids in your body. What about the most vital liquid of all. Is there acid in your blood?

The answer is "NO." The pH of blood is always between 7 and 7.4, meaning it is non-acid. If your blood ever fell below 7, death would come immediately. When you eat acid foods, your blood and digestive juices must neutralize the acid. Your body must borrow mineral salts, etc., from your blood and tissues to counteract the increased acidity.

Because basic properties are borrowed from the blood and tissues to combat the acids, you have robbed your tissues and they can begin to degenerate. Degeneration leads to dryness of tissues surrounding your joints, for example. Dryness leads to arthritic joints and the very disease we are trying to prevent.

To protect the blood—keep it from falling below the fatal level of 7—many organs throughout your body "donate" neutralizing salts. They give up their own minerals, even if they injure themselves by doing so. Your tissues make this sacrifice, at the risk of degenerating and becoming dry. The kidneys, lungs and liver all surrender parts of themselves to fight the acids.

Our purpose is to save our bodies from this terrible toll. We have warned you about fruit juices and certain liquids. Now, let's examine solid foods.

Fortunately, we can honestly tell you that most

meat, fish, cereals and vegetables do not disturb the "acidity level" in your body. All these foods are found in the menus recommended for arthritics later in this book.

Briefly, to defeat arthritis, we want to <u>eliminate</u> acids and <u>gain</u> oils.

Chapter XIV

Avoid Foods with the Wrong Oils

Much has been said favoring oils for arthritics. In the last chapter, for instance, we learned to keep acids away from the lubricating oils in our bodies— and why this is essential if we expect to recover from arthritis.

Most of this book has been urging you to add more oils to your system. Before anyone gains the impression that they should eat every oil-bearing food in sight, perhaps the time has come to remind you that there are "bad" oils, too.

To rid yourself of arthritis takes more than just eating chunks of fat. Such food can contain "wrong oils" which can clog your blood vessel "pipe-lines." This is worse than gaining no oils at all. If you select oily substances which are incorrect, they will do little except add to your weight, create excess energy (fat) or even lead to high blood pressure, gallbladder trouble or heart disease.

So, we must know how to differentiate between the very specific oils we need for lubrication and just any oil at all.

Here, just below, is a helpful chart which arthritics should consult to recognize the "wrong" oil in foods.

THE WRONG OILS (FOR ARTHRITICS)

All meat fats
(Eat lean meat instead!)

All vegetable oils

AVOID PARTICULARLY
  Bacon fat
  Cold cut meat fat
  Corned beef fat
  Ham fat
  Hamburg fat
  Lamb fat
  Pork chop fat
  Veal fat
  Lard

Any oil with sugar in it

AVOID PARTICULARLY
  Ice cream
  Chocolate candies

AVOID PARTICULARLY
  Almonds
  Brazil nuts
  Butternuts
  Cashews
  Chestnuts
  Cocoanut

AVOID PARTICULARLY
  All substitutes for butter
  Avocado oil
  Corn oil
  Cottonseed oil
  Olive oil
  Peanut butter
  Soya bean oil

● **MINERAL OIL**

  Filberts
  Hazel nuts
  Peanuts
  Pecans
  Pistachios
  Walnuts

Avoiding the oils in the foods listed above will play a deciding role in how long it will take an arthritic to become well.

Until now, most people probably thought that

oil is oil, good for energy only. Nothing could be farther from the truth.

Dr. P. Hawk is one expert who has done much to prove that all oils are not alike in their value to the body. In his book, *Practical Physiological Chemistry,* Dr. Hawk makes an outstanding contribution to medicine. Among other things, he says, in effect, THAT DIETARY OIL IS UNIQUE IN ITS POTENTIAL POSSIBILITIES <u>BECAUSE IT CAN BY-PASS THE LIVER</u>. We agree, and we will explain the importance of this fact to arthritics later, in Chapter XVIII.

The Right Oils, and How They Work for You

Having learned which oily foods to ignore, we will now go on to name the best foodstuffs. But just before we do, let us consult Dr. Hawk's findings on why <u>dietary</u> oils are good for you. He made the following points . . . we are restating now in our own words. . . .

WHAT THE RIGHT OILS WILL DO FOR YOUR BODY

1. Serve as a vehicle to introduce the oil-soluble vitamins, A, D, and E.
2. Influence the rate of calcification in bones and other tissues.
3. Aids in the digestion and absorption of other foods.

4. Repairs organic damage, as well as regenerating new tissues.

5. Carries vitamin K, the anti-hemorrhage substance, into the liver.

With all these benefits—the five described above, plus many more—all of us should seek out the right oil-bearing foods and make them a part of our daily diet.

Where can we find the correct oil ingredients? Here are six of the best sources, in the order of their effectiveness.

THE RIGHT OILS (FOR ARTHRITICS)

Cod liver oil
Milk
Eggs (soft boiled)
Butter
Certain fish (see page 65)
Cheddar cheese

The short size of this chapter should not mislead you. The past few paragraphs hold tremendous significance for your future. The conflict between right and wrong oils has bearing on more ailments than just arthritis. It is our firm belief that scientists, in years to come, will discover that oil deficiencies and oil tensions are factors in 80% of the diseases which kill mankind.

Why let your cells become disorganized, your blood vessels suffer occlusion, and general mayhem run wild in your body? Choose the right oils—they are so few in number—and practice common sense dietary habits.

AN ARTHRITIC'S MEALS MUST CONTAIN THE RIGHT KIND OF OIL

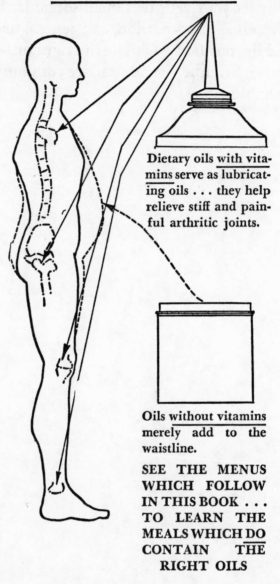

Dietary oils with vitamins serve as lubricating oils ... they help relieve stiff and painful arthritic joints.

Oils without vitamins merely add to the waistline.

SEE THE MENUS WHICH FOLLOW IN THIS BOOK ... TO LEARN THE MEALS WHICH DO CONTAIN THE RIGHT OILS

Chapter XV

Menus . . . Day by Day List of Correct Meals

Throughout this book we have stated that correct diet can help solve your arthritic problems. We have been examining specific foods, beverages and different oils. But, as yet, we have not put all these elements together into one meal. We need a complete menu—to show the proper quantities and the proper sequence of eating your food.

Here, then, in the following pages, are actual day by day lists—complete breakfasts, lunches and dinners—to serve as your guide.

These menus will start you toward recovery. Equally important, once you have gained relief, these diets will provide the essentials to <u>keep</u> you well. In the past, some treatments for arthritis have had merit. They have accomplished temporary results for the arthritic. Then—because a correct diet did not exist—the victim had a relapse. Now, such recurrence of pain can be prevented.

As we prepare to list daily menus we should take one other fact into consideration. The weight of each arthritic varies. Tall or small, stout or thin . . . these factors require changes in the amount of food you eat. You must maintain the average weight that is judged best for your build.

Therefore, in designing the menus which you are about to read, we carefully divided the meals into three categories. We show a typical week of foods recommended for arthritics of normal weight. Then, you will find a section of menus devoted to meals for the arthritic who is overweight. And, a third section for those who are underweight.

You know which section applies to you. Now ... refer to the next few pages ... and here's wishing you GOOD EATING! ...

SEVEN-DAY MENU—NORMAL WEIGHT

MONDAY

BREAKFAST

Whole wheat toast
   (buttered) ..... 2 slices
Egg .... 1 (soft boiled)
Stewed prunes
   or choice of melon in season
Milk .... 8 oz. glass

LUNCH

Whole wheat toast
   (buttered) ..... 1 slice
Fruit salad (sliced peaches, pears, apples, and cottage cheese on lettuce)
Milk .... 10 oz. glass

DINNER

Chicken broth ... ½ cup
Steak (lean) ...... Large serving
Asparagus .... ½ cup
Baked potato .... 1 (medium sized)
Milk .... 8 oz. glass

10 p.m.–11 p.m.
COD LIVER OIL MIXTURE
(Taken and mixed as described in Chapter XVII.)

TUESDAY

BREAKFAST

Oatmeal
   with milk ..... 1 cup
"Raw" wheat germ 2 tablespoons
   (mix into oatmeal when served)
Milk .... 8 oz. glass

LUNCH

Whole wheat
   or rye .... 1 roll
Butter .... 1 pat
Salad (shredded cabbage, green lettuce, grated carrot and cheese)
Milk .... 8 oz. glass

DINNER

Consommé
   clear .... 1 cup
Liver steak
   broiled .... 8 oz.
Steamed onions .. ½ cup
Spinach .... ½ cup
Green celery and lettuce salad
Milk .... 8 oz. glass

10 p.m.–11 p.m.
COD LIVER OIL MIXTURE

WEDNESDAY

BREAKFAST

Choice of bread (good grade)
   (buttered toast) 1 slice
Cottage cheese ... 1 cup
Several leaves of green lettuce
Wheat germ flake cereal
   (or some good-grade dry cereal like
   bran and fig or rice flake)
Milk .... 8 oz. glass

LUNCH

Tuna fish sandwich on whole
   wheat toast
Apple .... 1 large
Milk .... 8 oz. glass

DINNER

Roast beef (lean) Large serving
Green peas ...... ½ cup
Mashed potatoes . ½ cup
Carrots
Berries (in season) ½ cup
   or
Corn or bran muffin
Milk .... 8 oz. glass

10 p.m.–11 p.m.
COD LIVER OIL MIXTURE

THURSDAY

BREAKFAST

Oatmeal
   with milk ..... 1 cup
"Raw" wheat germ 2 tablespoons
Choice of black, unsulphured figs or
   stewed prunes
Milk .... 8 oz. glass

LUNCH

Vegetable soup .. 1 cup
Broiled lean hamburg on roll
Sliced raw onion (optional)
Milk .... ½ glass

DINNER

Lamb chops
   (lean) .... 2 medium
Mashed potatoes . ½ cup
String beans ..... ½ cup
Lettuce and tomato salad
Peaches .... 2 fresh
Milk .... 8 oz. glass

10 p.m.–11 p.m.
COD LIVER OIL MIXTURE

FRIDAY

BREAKFAST
Whole wheat toast 2 slices
Butter .... 1 pat
Egg (boiled) ..... 1 (3 minute)
Milk .... 8 oz. glass

LUNCH
Cheese sandwich (toasted)
Green lettuce and tomato slices,
Milk .... 8 oz. glass

DINNER
Broiled halibut .. Large slice
Cole slaw .... 1 cup
Lima beans
  (frozen) .... 1 cup
Apple
Milk .... 8 oz. glass

10 p.m.–11 p.m.
COD LIVER OIL MIXTURE

SATURDAY

BREAKFAST
Choice of dry cereal
Sliced banana
Cottage cheese ... ½ cup
Milk .... 8 oz. glass

LUNCH
Eggs on waffles ... 2 poached
(use corn muffin mix for waffles)
Celery
Milk .... 8 oz. glass

DINNER
Broiled steak
Baked potato
Cauliflower ..... 1 cup
Cucumber and celery salad
Melon (in season)
   or
Fruit cup (preferably fresh, if
  canned, drain syrup)
Milk .... 8 oz. glass

10 p.m.–11 p.m.
COD LIVER OIL MIXTURE

SUNDAY

BREAKFAST

Choice of fruit
  (see fruit list p. 150)
Corn muffins .... 2 (hot)
Butter .... 1 pat
Canadian bacon or ham (lean)
Eggs .... 2 (poached)
Milk .... 8 oz. glass

SUPPER

Cottage cheese ... Cup
Tossed salad
Apple
Milk .... 8 oz. glass

DINNER

Soup .... Cup
Roast chicken
Cranberry sauce
Sweet potato .... 1 medium sized
Brussel sprouts .. ½ cup
Celery
Milk .... 8 oz. glass

10 p.m.–11 p.m.
COD LIVER OIL MIXTURE

Special Facts to Remember

For persons of normal weight and height, experts say that you should consume foods which will give you approximately 2,200 calories per day. The menus you have just read offer between 1,900 and 2,200 calories daily. So, if you are still hungry after eating the meals described, you may adjust the menus upward.

In other words, you may eat larger portions of the foods . . . just eat them in the same order and the same type.

You will notice that citric fruits and all fruit juices have been eliminated from the breakfast meal. This is a major change for most people. It is necessary, however, because of their drying effect on the body.

Missing, too, from the menus is the usual glass of water placed with each meal. Arthritics should try to drink their entire daily supply of water at least one hour before breakfast—because it will then have a mildly laxative effect and will do no damage to dietary oils.

Probably you are pleased to notice the variety of enjoyable foods listed in the menus. And an even wider choice of pleasant fruits and vegetables suitable for arthritics can be found by turning ahead to pages 149–150.

Seven-Day Menu—Underweight Arthritics

If you are underweight, and you also have arthritis, you need to be doubly careful about your dietary habits. Select foods which will help you overcome both problems simultaneously. The menus on the next few pages will accomplish both purposes for you.

Meanwhile, however, along with eating the correct meals, you should take special note of the following facts:

1. Eat both cereal and eggs for breakfast every day.
2. Use butter on all hot vegetables.
3. Drink a 10-ounce glass of milk at every meal.
4. Eliminate all coffee-drinking.
5. Enjoy more soup, at more meals.
6. Eat meat frequently, in larger portions.
7. Drink an additional glass of milk one hour after eating your evening meal.

The above suggestions can be of basic aid to add weight healthfully.

Study the menus on the next pages. You will see that many oil-bearing foods are included. In many cases the same food item contains several types of oils. Some will add weight to your body, while other of the oils will nourish your joint linings. Both jobs will be done at the same time.

Here, Monday through Sunday, is the dietary plan for you.

SEVEN-DAY MENU—UNDERWEIGHT ARTHRITICS

MONDAY

BREAKFAST
Whole wheat toast
  (buttered) ..... 2 slices
Eggs (boiled) 2 (3-minute)
Stewed prunes
  or black, unsulphured figs
Milk .... 10 oz. giass

LUNCH
Bowl of chicken soup
Toasted cheese sandwich
Tossed salad
Milk .... 10 oz. glass

DINNER
Broiled chicken
Mashed potato ... ½ cup
Spinach .... 1 cup
Green celery ..... 4 stalks
Milk .... 10 oz. glass

7-7.30 p.m.
Milk .... 10 oz. glass

10 p.m.–11 p.m.
COD LIVER OIL MIXTURE

(Taken and mixed as described in
  Chapter XVII.)

TUESDAY

BREAKFAST
Pancakes; buckwheat
Butter .... 2 pats
Cottage cheese ... 1 cup
Milk .... 10 oz. glass

LUNCH
Whole wheat toast
(buttered) ..... 2 slices
Tuna fish salad
Tomato and cucumber slices
Lettuce
Apple
Milk .... 10 oz. glass

DINNER
Broiled liver and onions
Baked potato and butter
Steamed carrots
Green lettuce and tomato
Melon
Milk .... 10 oz. glass

7-7.30 p.m.
Milk .... 10 oz. glass

10 p.m.–11 p.m.
COD LIVER OIL MIXTURE

WEDNESDAY

BREAKFAST
Toast (buttered) . 1 slice
Dry cereal and banana
"Raw" wheat germ
(optional) ..... 2 tablespoons
Egg (boiled) 1 (3-minute)
Milk .... 10 oz. glass

LUNCH
Green pea soup .. 1 cup
Bologna sandwich on rye bread
(buttered)
Carrot and raisin salad
Milk .... 10 oz. glass

DINNER
Shrimp cocktail
Broiled lobster
Succotash .... 1 cup
Cranberry sauce
Fruit cup (apples, peaches, pears,
cherries) (preferably fresh)
Milk .... 10 oz. glass

7-7.30 p.m.
Milk .. .. 10 oz. glass

10 p.m.–11 p.m.
COD LIVER OIL MIXTURE

THURSDAY

BREAKFAST

Whole wheat toast
(buttered) ..... 1 slice
Egg .... 1 (poached)
Wheat cereal .... 1 cup
Milk .... 10 oz. glass

LUNCH

Cream cheese sandwich
Fruit salad
Milk .... 10 oz. glass

DINNER

Barley and bean
soup .... 1 cup
Squash .... 1 cup
Broccoli .... 1 cup
Celery and radishes
Banana
Milk .... 10 oz. glass

7–7.30 p.m.
Milk .... 10 oz. glass

10 p.m.–11 p.m.
COD LIVER OIL MIXTURE

FRIDAY

BREAKFAST

Whole wheat toast 2 slices
Butter .... 1 pat
Oatmeal .... 1 cup
"Raw" wheat germ 2 tablespoons
Milk .... 10 oz. glass

LUNCH

Crackers and butter
Bowl of tomato soup
Hot vegetable plate
Milk .... 10 oz. glass

DINNER

Broiled codfish
Lima beans
(frozen) .... 1 cup
Baked eggplant .. 1 cup
Lettuce, celery, tomato salad
Berries (in season) ½ cup
Milk .... 10 oz. glass

7–7.30 p.m.
Milk .... 10 oz. glass

10 p.m.–11 p.m.
COD LIVER OIL MIXTURE

SATURDAY

BREAKFAST

Rye toast and
   butter .... 2 slices
Eggs (boiled) 2 (3-minute)
Choice of melon or prunes (see fruit
   list p. 150)
Wheat germ flake cereal
   (or some good-grade dry cereal like
   bran and fig or rice flake)
Milk .... 10 oz. glass

LUNCH

Beef soup .... 1 cup
Frankfurt .... 1 on roll
Tossed salad
Milk .... 10 oz. glass

DINNER

Hamburg patties . 2 (broiled)
Potato .... 1 (baked)
String beans .. .. 1 cup
1 apple
Milk .... 10 oz. glass

7-7.30 p.m.

Milk .... 10 oz. glass

10 p.m.–11 p.m.

COD LIVER OIL MIXTURE

SUNDAY

BREAKFAST

Choice of bread (good-grade)
   (buttered toast) 1 slice
Egg .... 1 (poached)
Oatmeal .... ½ cup
"Raw" wheat germ 2 tablespoons
   (mix into oatmeal when served)
Milk .... 10 oz. glass

SUPPER

Vegetable soup .. 1 cup
Cottage cheese ... 1 cup
French toast ..... 2 slices
Banana
Milk .... 10 oz. glass

DINNER

Large steak
Salad of lettuce, tomato, cucumber,
   radishes, celery, carrots
Mashed potato ... ½ cup
Milk .... 10 oz. glass

7-7.30 p.m

Milk .... 10 oz. glass

10 p.m.–11 p.m.

COD LIVER OIL MIXTURE

Seven-Day Menu—Overweight Arthritics

If you are overweight, you have probably been told to avoid food with oils. They are supposed to be fattening. Yet, throughout this book, we have been telling arthritics that they must consume added amounts of oil to lubricate their joints.

How, then, can you be expected to follow a diet and keep to a menu which emphasizes oils? How can you keep from gaining weight, and still observe the plan which is outlined in this book?

There are two answers. First, the special menus we are going to list for you contain lubricating oils. There's a difference between lubricating oils and "energy" oils. Your choice of oils decides whether the oils will lubricate—or just serve as energy and fatten you. The difference is whether oils contain vitamins.

Secondly, the order in which you eat your food will determine what the oil does for your body. Adhere to these menus, eat specific oil-bearing foods in the proper sequence, and most of the oils will not turn to fat. They will be used to lubricate before they have a chance to become energy (fat).

For arthritics who are obese, employ this schedule. . . .

SEVEN-DAY MENU—OVERWEIGHT ARTHRITICS

MONDAY

BREAKFAST
Egg (boiled) 1 (3-minute)
Melba toast ......1 slice
Stewed prunes or black, unsulphured
  figs
Milk ....6 oz. glass

LUNCH
Fruit salad (peaches, apples, prunes,
  and cottage cheese)
Milk .... 6 oz. glass

DINNER
Vegetable soup .. 1 cup
Steak .... Large serving
Raw carrots ..... ½ cup
Broccoli .... ½ cup
Milk .... 6 oz. glass

10 p.m.–11 p.m.
COD LIVER OIL MIXTURE
(Taken and mixed as described in
  Chapter XVII.)

TUESDAY

BREAKFAST
Oatmeal ....½ cup
"Raw" wheat germ 1 to 2 tablespoons
  (mix into oatmeal when served)
Milk ....6 oz. glass

LUNCH
Vegetable salad (tomatoes, lettuce,
  celery, carrots, radishes, green pep-
  per, cucumber)
Small amount of mayonnaise
  (optional)
Whole wheat toast 1 slice
Milk .... 6 oz. glass

DINNER
Roast beef (lean
  and medium
  rare) .... Large portion
Corn .... ½ cup
Salad (green celery and lettuce)
Milk .... 6 oz. glass

10 p.m.–11 p.m.
COD LIVER OIL MIXTURE

WEDNESDAY

BREAKFAST
Wheat germ flake cereal with 4 oz.
  of milk
(or any good-grade dry cereal like
  bran and fig or rice flake)
Cottage cheese .... ½ cup
Milk .... ½ glass

LUNCH
Broiled hamburg on roll
Tossed salad
Milk .... 6 oz. glass

DINNER
Broiled salmon
Baked potato .... ½ (with jacket)
Green celery .... 2 stalks
Green peas ...... ½ cup
Milk .... 6 oz. glass

10 p.m.–11 p.m.
COD LIVER OIL MIXTURE

THURSDAY

BREAKFAST
Choice of bread
  (good grade)   1 slice
Butter .... ½ pat
Choice of fruit
  (see fruit list p. 150)
Milk .... 6 oz. glass

LUNCH
Sliced egg on lettuce
Tomato, celery, carrot salad
Melba toast ..... 2 pieces
Milk .... 6 oz. glass

DINNER
Bouillon .... 1 cup
Broiled liver
Cole slaw .... 1 cup
Succotash .... ½ cup
Milk .... 6 oz. glass

10 p.m.–11 p.m.
COD LIVER OIL MIXTURE

FRIDAY

BREAKFAST
Rye bread toasted 1 slice
Egg .... 1 (poached)
Milk .... 6 oz. glass

LUNCH
Cottage cheese ... 1 cup
Blueberries ...... ½ cup
Honeydew melon. 1 wedge
Milk .... 6 oz. glass

DINNER
Tuna fish salad
Carrot and raisin salad on lettuce
Eggplant .... ½ baked
Apple
Milk .... 6 oz. glass

10 p.m.–11 p.m.
COD LIVER OIL MIXTURE

SATURDAY

BREAKFAST
Choice of black, unsulphured figs or
    stewed prunes .2
Eggs .... 2 (poached)
Whole wheat toast 1 slice
Milk .... 6 oz. glass

LUNCH
Clear soup ...... 1 cup
Cold cut plate
Tossed salad
Milk .... 6 oz. glass

DINNER
Broiled hamburg patties
Cauliflower ..... ½ cup
Beets .... ½ cup
Tomato wedges
Milk .... 6 oz. glass

10 p.m.–11 p.m.
COD LIVER OIL MIXTURE

SUNDAY

BREAKFAST

Oatmeal .... ½ cup
"Raw" wheat germ 2 tablespoons
Milk .... 6 oz. glass

SUPPER

Cheese sandwich
Celery
Apple
Milk .... 6 oz. glass

DINNER

Chicken broth ... 1 cup
Broiled chicken
Lettuce and tomato salad
Brussel sprouts .. ½ cup
Cranberry sauce . 1 tablespoon
Milk .... 6 oz. glass

10 p.m.–11 p.m.
COD LIVER OIL MIXTURE

IMPORTANT REMINDER FOR ARTHRITICS OF ALL WEIGHTS

There is no law which says that you must take the cod liver oil mixture between 10 p.m. and 11 p.m. each night. You will notice that the 10 to 11 p.m. hour was listed in all of the menus on the preceding pages. . . . However, this hour was used merely because it is the approximate bedtime of many arthritics.

The point to remember is to drink the oil mixture at least four hours after your evening meal. (With the average dinner about 6 p.m., the 10 to 11 p.m. hour would apply.)

Adjust the time of taking the mixture to your own schedule. Just wait four hours after your evening meal, whatever time it ends. Then, when you retire, the oil will remain undisturbed while you sleep and will have a chance to be assimilated.

Quick Check List of Good Foods

Many nutritious and pleasant-tasting foods were included in the menus you have just read. Now, to give you even more variety—and still offer foods which are beneficial to arthritics—here are added items you may enjoy.

For easy reference, when you're making up your shopping list, use the following guide. . . .

You may substitute any of these foods and use them in any menu found in this book.

Foods Recommended for Arthritics

MEATS

Chicken	Lamb chops (lean)	Steak (sirloin, porterhouse, top round, filet mignon, T-bone)
Ham (lean)	Lamb, leg of (lean)	
Hamburg (lean)	Liver	
Heart (beef)	Pork (center cut, lean)	Tongue
Kidney	Roast beef (lean)	Turkey
		Veal

FISH

Bluefish	Halibut	Scallops
Butterfish	Lobster	Shrimp
Clams	Mackerel	Swordfish
Cod	Oyster	Tuna
Crab	Pompano	Trout
Flounder	Salmon	Whitefish

VEGETABLES

Asparagus	Chard	Onions
Beans	Corn	Peas
Beets	Cucumber	Peppers
Broccoli	Eggplant	Potatoes
Brussel sprouts	Endive	Radishes
Cabbage	Escarole	Spinach
Carrots	Lettuce	Squash
Cauliflower	Lima beans	String beans
Celery	Okra	Tomatoes

FRUITS

Apples	Cherries	Plums
Bananas	Crenshaw melon	Prunes
Blackberries	Figs	Raisins
Blueberries	Honeydew melon	Raspberries
Cantaloupe	Peaches	Strawberries
Casaba melon	Pears	

(When any of the above fruits come in canned form, *be sure to drain away and discard the syrup*.)

(The sugar, concentrated in the juices, is detrimental to arthritics.)

DAIRY PRODUCTS

CHEESES—American
        Blue cheese
        Cheddar
        Cottage
        Cream
        Swiss
EGGS
MILK—(Homogenized vitamin D)
      Raw milk, well shaken

BREADS

Bran or corn muffins
Brown bread
Corn bread
Cracked wheat bread
Graham or rye rolls
Pumpernickel
Rye
Whole wheat

Special Suggestions for your Plan of Eating

On the previous pages we have given you a comprehensive list of favorable foods. Now, however, there are some important facts every arthritic should remember about how and when to eat those foods. Here are some basic reminders. . . .

1. Watch the order in which you consume foods and liquids . . . follow the menus.

2. Men who follow the menus in this book may increase the amount of meats, fish, eggs, cheeses, and vegetables . . . just eat larger portions, if you're still hungry.

3. For a laxative, use 1 to 2 tablespoons of raw wheat germ on hot or cold breakfast cereal or a salad. Use it daily.

4. *Also as a mild laxative, drink a glass of warm water approximately 1 hour before breakfast.*

5. *If you are using any type of laxative, be sure to take it before breakfast.*

6. *If you use mineral oil, take it at least 2 hours before breakfast. Preferably not at all!*

7. *After a light dinner or supper, allow 2 or 3 hours before you take cod liver oil.*

8. *When meat is the main dinner course, allow 3 to 4 hours before taking cod liver oil.*

9. *Drink coffee, if you must, at least 10 to 30 minutes before any meal. Never with or right after a meal. Wait 3 to 4 hours.*

10. *Use saccharin or a sugar substitute for sweetening coffee.*

11. *Use a minimum of salt on your food . . . it can lead to constipation.*

12. *Use butter to broil meats, whenever possible. Broil meats until they are medium rare. Trim away all fats.*

13. *Eat liver and beef steak frequently.*

14. *In the menus, the term "large portion" of meat or fish means an 8 oz. serving—the weight as it is served.*

15. *Eat generous amounts of tossed salad, made from green lettuce leaves together with green celery and raw cabbage. Sour cream, yogurt or minimal amounts of your favorite dressing may be used as salad dressings.*

16. *Should you have colitis it is advisable to pressure-cook raw fruits and vegetables briefly. This may also apply to those having difficulty masticating because of dentures.*

17. *Avoid the use of sweets. (Sugar, candy,*

*preserves, syrups, molasses, honey—either by them-
selves or on foods.)*

*18. Beware of anything sour. (Vinegar, lemon
or lemon juice, grapefruit, or grapefruit juice,
grapes, or similar fruits.)*

*19. Try not to use any vegetable oils or animal
greases . . . such as oleomargarine, olive oil, lard,
etc.*

*20. Remove the fat from meats before cook-
ing.*

*21. Avoid eating farina, grits, or bleached
cereals.*

The menus in this chapter really get results for
arthritics. Each and every menu has been carefully
tested, tried and proven successful. They were developed in kitchens and laboratories to provide you
with the essential oils your body needs to give you
better health. Use these menus, as your daily guide.

EATING FOODS IN THE PROPER ORDER . . .

Throughout this book—and in all menus—you will notice instruc-
tions suggesting that foods be eaten "in the following order."

The term, "in the following order" does not mean that each food
must be eaten separately and consumed in its entirety before the next
food is eaten. You may eat one type of food, and then eat any other
item of food on your plate . . . just avoid the chronic mistake of
drinking water or wrong liquids in the midst of the meal.

If you wish, you may substitute foods in any menu—selecting
from the lists on pages 149 and 150—merely avoid drinking the wrong
liquids while eating.

Chapter XVI

Can Vitamins Speed Relief?

The title of this chapter asks a question. Medical authorities have several answers on whether vitamins can help affect arthritis. Let's see what they say. . . .

A Disease of the Constitution

Most arthritis, in the opinion of many outstanding rheumatologists, is a constitutional disease, which means, prior to the start of arthritis—or while it is in progress—other parts of the body can be simultaneously diseased. Vitamin deficiencies are present, too, but are not necessarily directly connected with the arthritis.

Dr. R. H. Freyberg, in a report in the *Journal of the American Medical Association* (August 8, 1942), summed up the relationship between vitamins and arthritis. He said, in effect, that there was no relationship in the case of most vitamins to arthritis proper. But one vitamin—vitamin D—was allowed a supporting role.

The point was established that vitamin A deficiencies were not uncommon among people who had arthritis and rheumatic diseases. However, when the vitamin deficiencies were corrected, the arthritis still remained. This also held true in the case of other vitamins, like vitamin B. (Arthritics are frequently deficient in vitamin B, as manifested by constipation.) Again, though, correcting the constipation by means of vitamin B does not correct the arthritis.

As was stated earlier, leading doctors do believe that one vitamin can play a supporting role in the fight against arthritis. Vitamin D.

So, let's explore vitamin D. You, as an arthritic, should know whether you have a vitamin D deficiency. You should learn to recognize the symptoms . . . so you can take steps to correct the trouble. Here is a check list, do you have any of these signs. . . .

Vitamin D

Deficiency Symptoms Include

Rickets
Enlarged joints
Bow legs
Tendency to tooth decay
Soft brittle bones
Curved spine
Retarded growth
Jutting jaws—poor facial contour
Brittle, splitting nails.

The next question, quite logically, is how to correct these conditions. What foods will give your body added amounts of vitamin D? Here is a helpful chart. . . .

Foods Which Are a Good Source of Vitamin D

Beefsteak, lean	Halibut
Butter	Herring
Cheddar cheese	Liver
Clams	Mackerel
Cod liver oil	Salmon
Cream	Sardines
Egg yolk	Shrimp
Halibut liver oil	Tuna
Vitamin D milk	

Above, we have listed some foods which contain the right vitamin for arthritics. Now, what about obtaining vitamins the so-called "easy way"? Will vitamin pills or tablets do the trick?

In one word, the answer is "No!" My tests and research indicate that taking vitamins in concentrated form (capsules, etc.) does not gain the best results. At least not for victims of rheumatic diseases.

If you disagree, then swallow vitamin capsules daily. But take them with MILK. They may not harm you, they just don't contribute particularly to your war on arthritis.

Meanwhile, however, food and diet can bring you greater amounts of vitamins. Drink milk at every meal. Take cod liver oil (containing vitamin D) until you have normally lustrous skin, scalp and hair. Eat green leafy vegetables, whole grain bread, soups, and lean meats (like broiled steak, liver and roast beef). Then, you will not even require multiple vitamin tablets.

The only reason to take special preparations of vitamins (drugstore variety) is if you really feel that your daily diet of foods is deficient. If you are unable to obtain or eat the correct foods, then you can supplement your diet with vitamins from bottles.

Dr. T. Spies of the Hillman Nutrition Clinic in Birmingham, Alabama, feels that it would be safer for people to take multiple vitamins not knowing whether you need them, rather than trying to run your bodies on depleted foods. That's the safe way.

Dr. Spies is an internationally known and respected nutritionist, and we happen to agree with him.

This chapter has covered vitamins and their affect on arthritis. Summed up, they are valuable to your general health. But only vitamin D will directly help arthritics. And, it must be taken in oil form, <u>not</u> in concentrated capsules or tablets. Other chapters in this book will give you additional information on how to increase your vitamin D supply.

ALL MACHINES NEED SPECIAL TYPES OF OIL . . .
To lubricate bearings and "joints"

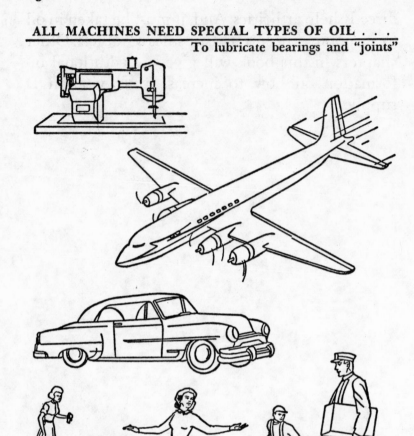

INCLUDING THE MACHINERY OF THE HUMAN BODY

The next chapter tells the best type of oil to lubricate stiffened arthritic joints. Oil away your stiffness and pain . . .

Chapter XVII

Cod Liver Oil Is a Key Weapon

Since we have agreed that vitamin D is an essential needed to defeat our arthritis, we should now look for the fastest way to secure the vitamin for our bodies.

The quickest, safest and most certain method to obtain vitamin D is to take cod liver oil. Yes, plain old-fashioned cod liver oil is our key weapon. This may sound strange and surprising to you. But to prove our point, let us examine the opinions of several leading doctors who also agree on the value of this oil.

One brilliant piece of arthritis research with cod liver oil was done by Dr. Ralph Pemberton of Pennsylvania. In the *Archives of Internal Medicine* (as far back as March, 1920), Dr. Pemberton wrote his "Studies on Arthritis in the Army, Based on 400 Cases." In case after case, he described the improvement which his soldier patients experienced when given cod liver oil. He found it effective if his patients were kept away from "inferior-type" starches.

One of Dr. Pemberton's later books, *The Medical and Orthopedic Management of Chronic*

Arthritis (1935), is a classic. It, too, reported favorably on cod liver oil.

Going back even farther we find physicians more than 100 years ago who were already on the righ track concerning cod liver oil. A book by Dr. L. J. de Jongh, called *Cod Liver Oil* and published in 1849, makes one of the early references to its use for chronic rheumatism.

In the book, Dr. de Jongh gives a list of twenty doctors and summarizes their feelings about the tremendous value of cod liver oil for arthritic conditions. THEY ALL AGREED IN THEIR OPINION THAT COD LIVER OIL IN THE TREATMENT OF CHRONIC ARTHRITIS WAS SUPERIOR TO ANY OTHER METHOD EVER DEVISED. The findings of these doctors were made by actually using cod liver oil in treating their rheumatic patients. The oil was successful for their patients, where everything else had failed.

To digress for a moment, it is interesting to note that cod liver oil has value in many other fields of medicine, too. It has been used for anemia and even as an aid in pregnancy.

A report from Dr. H. Berglund was published in the *Proceedings of the Society for Experimental Biology and Medicine,* under the title "Deficiency Anemia in Chinese, Responding to Cod Liver Oil." In this report Dr. Berglund told of research done during a famine in northern China. The victims had diets which were low on fat and on the verge of an oil-soluble vitamin deficiency.

After severe bouts with diarrhea, many Chinese developed anemia and tissue swelling. Feeding them a liver diet had no effect on the anemia. It was the same kind of anemia found among pregnant women when their diet was insufficient. Iron supplement could not control this type of anemia.

Cod Liver Oil to the Rescue

Imagine the satisfaction among these researchers when they suddenly discovered that by giving cod liver oil for only two months, they corrected the anemia!

As for pregnancy, with or without anemia, research on oil-free diets was started by experimenting with rats in the year 1929. Experts found that as the oil deficiency progressed, ovulating cycles became longer and longer and the litters were being lost. When rats were given cod liver oil, their ovulation cycle was not impaired and they bore normal litters.

Does this bear any relation to the female arthritic of the human species? Many arthritic mothers suddenly become well during pregnancy? Why? Perhaps their good fortune is the result of drinking more milk during pregnancy. Then, too, more women—whether they have arthritis or not—are advised during motherhood to take cod liver oil.

This oil is unique as "baby insurance." It helps prevent miscarriage by stocking the woman's body with iodine. This means the thyroid-ovary cycle is not impaired as easily.

Perhaps miscarriage in female arthritics is not just accidental, but results from the tremendous demand for iodine which is literally stolen from the ovaries for metabolic reasons.

Still another disease that has been treated with cod liver oil is tuberculosis. Dr. H. E. Kirschner reported success in this field. He is the physician who wrote the Foreword appearing in the front of this book. (Again, at this point, may I express my sincere appreciation for his contributing his opinions about my work.)

Returning to the subject of cod liver oil and its advantages for arthritics, we have now cited several examples of doctors who believe in its effectiveness. Earlier in the book, you have read a description of symptoms which prove that arthritis is an oil deficiency and a lack of vitamin D.

Check your own symptoms of dryness. Think about them, and think about the evidence you have read. Perhaps by now you agree that you do need oil-soluble vitamin D.

Ready to take cod liver oil? Fine. There is only one more fact you should know. For maximum effectiveness, the oil should be consumed in the proper quantity at the proper time of day.

In other words, there should be a definite way to take the oil. A set of rules. In a moment, we will list the rules and give you an exact guide.

To add even more value to the cod liver oil, we have developed a process whereby it can be emulsified with orange juice. When we combine the oil with orange juice, the entire mixture is more easily assimilated—it travels more readily from the stomach into the bloodstream and reaches arthritic joints in greater supply.

THE RULES

HERE IS YOUR BLUEPRINT TO HEALTH

FOR BEST RESULTS TAKE THE EMULSION OF COD LIVER OIL AND ORANGE JUICE JUST BEFORE BEDTIME—AT LEAST 3 TO 4 HOURS AFTER YOUR EVENING MEAL. IF YOU PREFER TO RETIRE EARLY, THEN TAKE THE MIXTURE IN THE MORNING—1 TO 2 HOURS BEFORE BREAKFAST. THIS IS OPTIONAL. LET YOUR ARTERIES SERVE AS "OIL PIPELINES" FROM YOUR EMPTY STOMACH.

HOW TO MIX AND EMULSIFY THE ORANGE JUICE AND OIL

You will need an orange, some cod liver oil, a tablespoon, a juice strainer and two glasses, holding four ounces each.

1. Take one half (½) of a medium sized orange at room temperature and squeeze out the juice.

2. Strain the orange juice into a four ounce glass. Make certain that all pulp is removed.

3. Put two ounces of this strained orange juice into another four ounce glass (Glass No. 2). Discard any juice left over in Glass No. 1.

4. Add one tablespoon of pure cod liver oil to the Glass No. 2 which now contains the orange juice. (Use mint-flavored or wild cherry cod liver oil, if you wish, for a more pleasant taste.)

5. Stir well for 10 to 15 seconds. You will notice hundreds of tiny oil bubbles.

6. Pour the mixed oil and orange juice in Glass No. 2 back and forth, from one glass into the other, about 20 times. (Like someone mixing a Bromo Seltzer.) Many thousands of minute bubbles will now appear on the surface of the mixture.

7. Drink the mixture immediately.

8. Do not disturb this oil with food or water for at least four hours, if mixture is taken at night. If oil is taken in morning, 1 to 2 hours will be enough since stomach empties quicker under these conditions. (The body will retain the approximate 0.02% of organic iodine in the cod liver oil more successfully by pre-fasting and post-fasting routine.)

9. Take cod liver oil alone, without the orange juice, if you wish. It has some advantages without the juice, particularly if you have arthritis in its advanced stages. (If you are deformed, for example, you may take the oil by itself or mix it with 2 tbsp. of "cool milk." Usually the deformed stage of arthritis indicates an allergy to the citric acid or fruit sugar in the orange. After several months of straight oil, or oil and milk combination, you may then use a small amount of juice to mix the oil. Those who have not been ill too long—and are less sensitive to fruit juice— can use up to four tablespoons of strained orange juice. But no one should use more than four tablespoons of juice with the oil.

10. Keep your bottle of cod liver oil refrigerated at all times —to keep it from getting rancid. Also keep it out of sunlight.

11. It is important to use two small four ounce glasses to mix the ingredients. If we used a larger glass, more of the oil would be left clinging to the inside surface of the glass—and our bodies would get lesser amounts.

12. DO NOT MIX THE COD LIVER OIL IN LEMON OR GRAPEFRUIT JUICE. These juices are too caustic to use. Orange juice or cool milk is the *only* kind of liquid for our mixing purpose.

13. If a person has an ulcer in the stomach or has colitis— then mix the oil with 2-4 tbsp. cool milk. Or take oil by itself.

14. Do not use concentrated orange juice. It should be fresh, and put through a strainer.

15. Do not use cod liver oil capsules in place of bottled oil. The contents of capsules are quickly captured by the liver and the joint linings are cheated. If the gallbladder is removed a person can still take the pure cod liver oil. By emulsifying the oil with a correct liquid like orange juice or milk, the function of a healthy gallbladder is not needed since its purpose is merely to emulsify oils.

16. After a certain period of time, you should start to taper down on the use of cod liver oil mixture. When? Cut down after you see that any dryness of the hair or scalp has been

corrected. When a normal supply of wax returns to your ears. When your pain has been relieved is a good sign to ease up on the cod liver oil intake. Look for skin improvement.

However, do not stop suddenly . . . keep taking the mixture every other night, instead of daily. Continue to follow this plan for approximately three months. Then, use the oil at least twice a month indefinitely.

The above rules on how and when to take the cod liver oil mixture apply to millions of arthritics. To people with either osteo or rheumatoid arthritis, to cases which are in the early stages, moderately advanced and even the chronic cases. This cod liver oil lubricating plan has already been used successfully by thousands of arthritics, and it offers the best hope for the future.

The only exceptions—the only people who should deviate from the above rules—are those arthritics who simultaneously have certain additional diseases. For them, here are some special suggestions:

If you have arthritis and you are also suffering from gallbladder trouble, diabetes, high blood pressure or heart disease, mix the cod liver oil with the orange juice more thoroughly. Use the same two tablespoons of orange juice, but pour the solution back and forth between the two glasses at least 40 times, instead of 20 times. Because such people find that their bodies will not assimilate oils quite as quickly, they should take the cod liver oil every other night or just twice a week.

166

HOW TO HELP LUBRICATE ARTHRITIC JOINTS

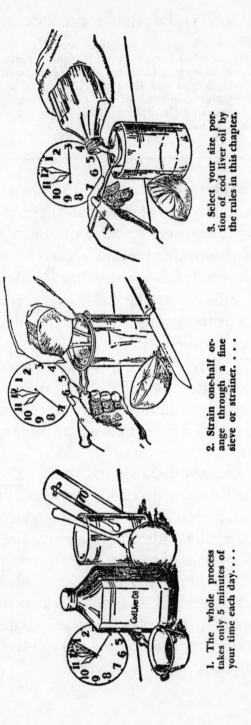

1. The whole process takes only 5 minutes of your time each day. . . .

2. Strain one-half orange through a fine sieve or strainer. . . .

3. Select your size portion of cod liver oil by the rules in this chapter.

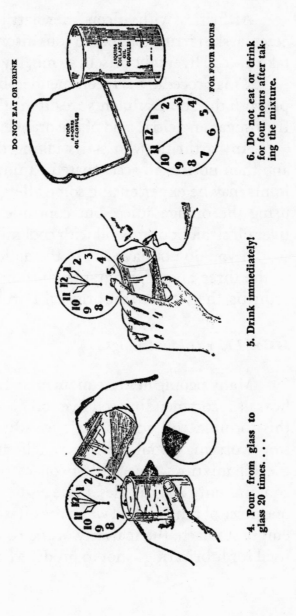

DO NOT EAT OR DRINK

FOOD ABSORBS OIL GLOBULES

LIQUIDS COLLECT OIL GLOBULES

FOR FOUR HOURS

6. Do not eat or drink for four hours after taking the mixture.

5. Drink immediately!

4. Pour from glass to glass 20 times. . . .

Arthritics with ulcers, dermatitis, psoriasis, eczema, skin irritations or nervous disorders should take the cod liver oil by itself, or mix it with milk.

This procedure is recommended because people with the above ailments are often allergic to the fruit sugar and citric acid of the orange.

Any arthritic who starts taking the mixture and then notices an accentuated pain in any of his joints may be experiencing some allergy. Just stop using the orange juice, but continue taking cod liver oil straight or mix oil with cool milk.

If you do not have any of the afflictions listed in the three above paragraphs to complicate your arthritis, then stick to the original 16 rules.

Is Cod Liver Oil Fattening?

Many people hesitate momentarily when they hear us recommending cod liver oil. They fear that this formula will add to their waistline. You can stop worrying about gaining weight from taking the oil mixture. One tablespoon of cod liver oil contains only 100 calories. (The equivalent of just one piece of candy.) And when the oil is taken on an empty stomach, the majority of the cod liver oil is used for lubricating—not to produce energy or fat.

SPECIAL COD LIVER OIL MIXING INSTRUCTIONS FOR ADVANCED CASES OF RHEUMATOID ARTHRITIS

People who have rheumatoid arthritis in the advanced stages may be sensitive (or allergic) to the citric acid and fruit sugar in orange juice. Therefore, these arthritics may mix the cod liver oil with 2 tablespoons of homogenized *milk* (at 60° to 70° F., cool) instead of using orange juice.

In fact, any arthritic who is allergic to orange juice may use milk with the cod liver oil.

For mixing and emulsifying cod liver oil—with either milk or orange juice—there is a second method, which is entirely suitable. Instead of using the utensils described on pages 166 and 167, you may place both ingredients in one 2-ounce jar, and shake vigorously . . . as illustrated below. . . .

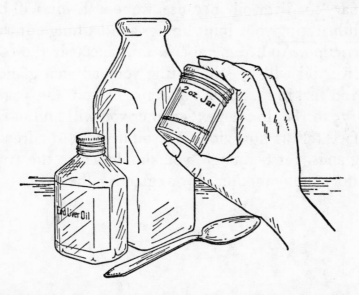

Second Approved Method to Mix and Emulsify Cod Liver Oil With Milk Or Orange Juice. Use the Same Ingredients: 1 Tablespoon of Cod Liver Oil and 2 Tablespoons of Cool Milk or *Strained* Orange Juice. (Read added facts in the Box above, on this Page.)

Where To Expect Relief

In most cases of arthritis, the first signs of improvement after taking cod liver oil will be noticed in the shoulders and hands. Pain, stiffness and swelling will start to recede—usually in that order. Next, you will feel relief in your knees and ankles. Finally, more motion will be restored to your hips and back. Pain-free motion!

Why will you gain all these benefits from ordinary cod liver oil? Because, we repeat, you will be lubricating your joint linings and bathing out the friction. And, remember, simultaneously the cod liver oil will be stimulating your adrenal glands and making natural cortisone for you. On pages 179 to 180, in the next chapter you will find more facts telling how vitamin D oil helps your adrenal glands. First, though, you should know the true story about another of your glands—the liver.

Chapter XVIII

Your Liver Can Cheat You

"Whether life is worth living depends on the liver!" That's an old expression which has been handed down through the years . . . and it has a great deal of truth in it.

Dr. H. A. Rafsky made popular another expression. Recently, he said, in effect: WE ARE NOT AS OLD AS OUR ARTERIES, BUT AS OLD AS OUR LIVERS!

Too many of us do not give our livers a second thought. Day after day, the organ performs a great job. But the liver can cheat an arthritic very badly —unless we know how to eat and drink properly!

Because the liver is so vital to your health, you should know all you can about this organ. . . .

The Liver

Reddish brown in color—and weighing on the average 1700 grams (3½ pounds)—the liver is situated to the right of the stomach and astride the small intestine.

Like every organ in the body, the liver has

duties that are varied and complex. Here is a summary of what the liver does:

1. Involved in maintaining water balance in the body.
2. Formation and secretion of bile.
3. Involved in antibody formation.
4. Deals with blood formation.
5. Concerned with acid-base balance.
6. Detoxifies foreign organic compounds.
7. Concerned with some hormones.
8. Deals with enzyme action.
9. Participation in vitamin metabolism.
10. Metabolism of inorganic salts, carbohydrates, protein compounds.
11. And extremely important to arthritics— metabolism of oils!

So, now you can see why the liver is referred to as the pantry of the human anatomy.

More than 500 different chemical actions are known to take place in this gland. All this activity is fostered by the location of the liver, which gives it first choice of just about everything you eat.

Serving, as it does, as the gateway to circulation within our body, the liver can gobble up the choicest particles of our food—without any protest from the rest of our anatomy.

The exception to this dictatorship by the liver is dietary oil.

Any oil leaving your stomach does not necessarily have to enter this toll gate known as the liver.
The oil does have an opportunity to by-pass the
greedy liver.

It is this chance to shuttle oils around the liver
that arthritics should take advantage of. Certainly
one organ should not be allowed to benefit at the
expense of adding to our arthritis pains. If we have
the common sense to maintain good eating habits,
we can have healthy livers—and healthy cartilages
and joint linings as well.

Here's how. How to get oils past the liver . . .
so they can lubricate arthritic joints. . . .

Eating Properly To Satisfy the Liver

When we eat rich foods like cake, pie, and ice
cream, the digestive system breaks the food down
into very fine sugar-like particles (glucose). These
are carried by a vein, called the portal vein, to the
liver. Liver cells decide whether the organ will utilize or store the glucose. When we overdo sweets or
starchy food, the liver must work harder to keep the
amount of sugar in our blood at a healthy level.

Researchers on arthritis have found that the
liver of a great many arthritics is extended by this
effort. The liver cannot throw off sugar for energy
utilization as quickly for arthritics and diabetics as
it does for people without these disorders.

Protein, too, must be forwarded through the liver.

Protein is to be found in lean meat, fish, and dairy products. Most protein—after it is broken down into its by-products—is shuttled to the liver. Here the by-products are subjected to the liver's fancy.

The liver cells decide whether to store the protein, or send it into the blood stream.

My research indicates that a person with arthritis should be on a high protein diet.

A Rich Liver Means Poor Joints

Just as in the case of proteins, the liver grabs up carbohydrates, minerals and vitamins. Because it is first in line, the liver takes everything it needs from food and becomes healthy—at the expense of the rest of our body. No wonder the liver can regenerate up to 75% of itself, being the only gland which can practically rebuild itself, if need be.

But, as arthritics, we are not interested in repairing the liver . . . we are concerned with regenerating joint linings and cartilage. What foods and materials can we use?

While the lining or cartilage of an arthritic joint is in the early stages of becoming worn, any repair substance escaping past the liver will be of great help. Again, the best substance to dodge the liver is our friend <u>cod liver oil</u>.

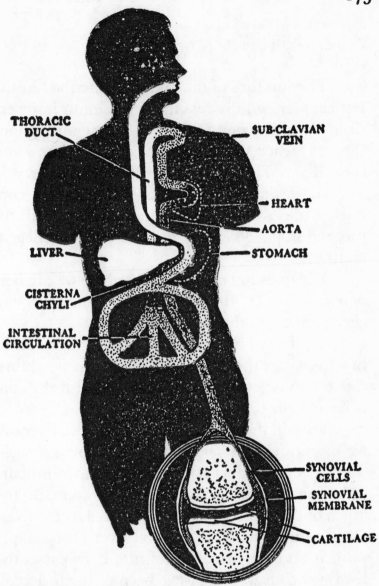

THORACIC DUCT

SUB-CLAVIAN VEIN

HEART

AORTA

LIVER

STOMACH

CISTERNA CHYLI

INTESTINAL CIRCULATION

SYNOVIAL CELLS

SYNOVIAL MEMBRANE

CARTILAGE

Cod liver oil—if taken properly—can by-pass the liver and stimulate the adrenal cortex. This activity will produce NATURAL CORTISONE of better quality . . . and the oils will travel all the way to your joints to lubricate and relieve arthritis!

Cod Liver Oil Can Build New Tissue

The mixture of oil, taken as described in the last chapter, will by-pass the liver almost in its entirety. It will go on to build new tissue throughout the body wherever it is needed. Doctors know and agree that cod liver oil has tissue-building power.

Dr. I. Smedley-MacClean, for instance, conducted tests which proved cod liver oil rebuilt tissue, and stopped kidneys, ovaries, etc., from degenerating.

The question now arises as to how we can best deliver this oil to the joint linings and cartilage to check osteo and rheumatoid arthritis.

Or, if need be, so it can fill the sac with oil in bursitis, cover the nerve with oil in neuritis, lubricate the muscles in myositis, and nourish the connective tissue in fibrositis.

To gain the fastest benefits from cod liver oil, we repeat, it must be taken on an empty stomach. To empty your stomach requires three to four hours of fasting. If there is any food in the stomach, too much of the cod liver oil will be seized by the liver. On an empty stomach, the cod liver oil is simply pushed on to the small intestine. It by-passes the liver, which is what we have been trying to accomplish.

The major reason for mixing cod liver oil with orange juice or cool milk is to defeat the liver. An emulsified mixture with orange juice or cool milk cheats the liver, beats it at its own game.

When we "sneak" the oil past the liver, we also gain added benefit from the iodine in cod liver oil.

Organic iodine is of tremendous value to arthritics. Dr. E. R. Eaton in the *Journal of the American Institute of Homeopathy* (March, 1941) lists the many accomplishments of iodine in the bloodstream:

1. Tends to "loosen" fibrous tissue.
   (Arthritics with stiff joints have fibrous tissue which can certainly stand "loosening.")
2. Iodine stimulates metabolism.
   (More than 30% of arthritics have a slightly lower than average basal metabolism.)
3. Dilates the blood vessels.
   (The rheumatoid arthritic often needs blood vessel dilation.)
4. Helps in the formation of hemoglobin.
   (The anemic rheumatoid can definitely use this property.)
5. Improves circulation.
   (Arthritics frequently need better circulation, when they have clammy, tingling or numbness in hands and feet.)

6. Helps correct uric acid metabolism.
   (Gouty arthritics need this form of help.)
7. Diminishes fatigue.
   (Which is a common problem of the rheu·
   matoid arthritic.)

The above seven services of iodine are added reasons why we should take cod liver oil. To gain iodine!

There are only 25 milligrams of iodine in our entire body. In other words, our whole supply could be placed on the head of a small common pin. About 60% of this is tied up by the thyroid gland. No wonder we need all the iodine we can get from our diet.

In a random sampling of cartilages from human beings—ages 20 through 95—Dr. W. Bauer and others found the cartilage was progressively wearing out. Certainly the cartilage wears out; it was probably losing its elasticity. The oils which could feed iodine to the joint fluid were missing from the diet!

We agree that the cartilage has no blood vessels, but cartilage can still take nourishment throughout its life by means of osmosis.

This filter-exchange process of osmosis is of no use, however, if the very substance the cartilage needs—a trace of iodine—is missing from the oil.

If the liver captures the iodine first, the cartilage suffers the loss.

Stimulate Your Adrenal Glands

We have been discussing the "robber-bandit" gland known as the liver. Another set of glands— the adrenals—also serve a vital function for arthritics. We should know more about them.

The adrenals are situated directly over the kidneys. Their purpose is to produce many different hormones. Hormones are substances which can be manufactured by glands through internal secretion if the specific gland is stimulated by a specific vitamin.

In the case of the adrenal glands, vitamin D in oil form is the only vitamin which can cause the manufacture of natural cortisone. Yes, the adrenals can make their own cortisone for your body. It is a hormone . . . one of 28 kinds inside the adrenals. When cortisone is released into the bloodstream, it travels into joint and connective tissues. These joint linings need the cortisone to add stickiness in and around the joints.

Now you know the main value of cortisone. It adds viscosity (sticky quality) to joint membranes. If you have brought lubricating oils to your joints by other means (cod liver oil, etc.) cortisone keeps the oil from seeping out of the tissues.

Rushing in Vitamin D, the Wrong Way

If we can make our own cortisone—by stimulating our adrenal glands with vitamin D—and gain so many other benefits from this vitamin, we might be inclined to rush around taking vitamin D pills or any other "fast way" to pile up a supply. Slow down, accept a word of warning.

There is no super-speed method to build up your store of vitamin D. Rushing overdoses into your system, in tablet or capsule form, can be dangerous. To prove it, let us examine the findings of Doctors I. Dreyer and C. I. Reed, as published in the *Archives of Physical Therapy*.

As doctors and allergists, Dreyer and Reed were treating two hay fever patients (who also had arthritis) with concentrated vitamin D in tablets. One of them found she could remove her ring from a swollen hand for the first time in years. The other discovered shoes getting loose on swollen feet. The beneficial effect was attributed to the vitamin D. And the cases apparently improved more by increasing the units of the vitamin.

Shortly after these two successes were reported (Volume 16, 1935) the United States became the scene of vitamin D hysteria. Doses of the vitamin were raised to 1,000,000 units daily—for each arthritic patient as well as for hay fever victims. Before long it was found that the human body could be expected to take only so much vitamin D. Then, the body began to rebel against this crystalline form of the vitamin. In many cases these overdose tablets proved toxic to the kidneys.

In 1939, after a series of deaths as a result of vitamin D auto-intoxication, the Council of Pharmacology and Chemistry discredited the use of massive doses of vitamin D in tablets or capsules for arthritis.

This incident left a bad impression in the minds of the American medical profession. Many doctors still believe today that their patients can be harmed by overdoses of vitamin D. Overdosage will occur, however, only by the excessive intake of vitamin D CONCENTRATES made up into TABLETS OR CAPSULES.

There is no danger from the amount of vitamin D in cod liver oil. Many tablets have more than 300,000 units of vitamin D in each dose.

By using pure cod liver oil daily—at 1,000 units per dose (as described in our rules on pages 163 to 165)—it would take nearly a full year to equal the units in one crystalline tablet.

Medical Authorities Agree About the Liver

Perhaps, now that the facts about your liver have been explained to you, the whole theme of this book may make more sense. Your own common sense will now tell you that lubricating oils are desperately needed by an arthritic body and they must be able to shuttle past your liver. Many outstanding doctors agree that the liver is deeply involved with oil metabolism. We would like to cite just two more cases. . . .

Dr. A. C. Frazer, in the *Journal of Physiology* (Volume 103, 1944–45), showed how oil, if emulsified, can be drawn primarily into the lymphatic system. This is the system of pipelines which leads more directly to the joints. Stated simply, this means that you can prevent more oils from entering the liver just by mixing them into an emulsifying liquid or agent, like orange juice.

If you want to do some further reading on this important aspect of your arthritic recovery program, may we suggest a report written by Dr. A. White. It can be found in a book entitled *Diseases of the Metabolism* (published by W. B. Saunders, Philadelphia, 1947). Dr. White contributed a whole chapter on lipid (oil) metabolism.

As this chapter has proven, dietary oils to aid the arthritic can enter the body by only two routes. Either through the liver, or around it. You can decide the course . . . by following our suggested rules.

Having explored all the difficulties caused by our liver, let's face up to another serious complication which threatens arthritics. Constipation. There's a whole chapter on this menace, just ahead.

Chapter XIX

How Constipation Affects Arthritics

Constipation often accompanies arthritis. It complicates the disease, and makes plans of dieting more difficult to follow. So, let us examine the whole problem of constipation.

Let me give you more knowledge on the subject—and the answers to some of your questions.

The need for having regular bowel habits is something parents impress upon their children at an early age. Ironically, most often it is the teaching parent who is <u>not regular</u>. The parents, along with millions of adults, try to use drugs or other laxative fads of the day.

The Lemon Juice Craze

One favorite method of trying to keep regular is to dilute the juice of a lemon with a glass of water. This myth goes back several hundred years. In 1950, however, reports began appearing in the medical and dental journals showing how teeth were being etched by the citric acid of lemon juice.

Warnings are now issued that people with arthritis should be on guard against lemon or diluted lemon juice as a laxative measure.

Please avoid the lemon habit—in spite of the fact that it is effective as a laxative. The citric acid of lemon juice is definitely able to stimulate muscle contractions. Instead, if you must, use citrate of magnesia. This employs the same evacuating principle, without drying out your body.

Warm Water Before Breakfast

A pre-breakfast drink of warm water is supposed to act as a laxative. It works, too. But when taken in the morning, be sure it's at least one hour before breakfast. Water taken by itself does have a beneficial action on sluggish bowels. It may be slower, without the lemon, but it is by far the better way. There will be absolutely no harmful side effects, like drying out the system.

While water in the morning is helpful, water during the day works against bowel regularity. Once you start eating, the process of digestion takes hours. Flooding your stomach with water during the day will only defeat proper digestion.

Mineral Oil

Crude mineral oil was discovered by the Indians on top of stagnant water in the oil fields. Today, mineral oil is refined into pure form from petroleum.

Refineries could not sell mineral oil for automobile use, so their representatives educate people to pour it into their bodies. Just the way mineral oil does not pass qualifications for a car carburetor, it forms puddles of useless oil in your intestinal loops. This finding was published recently in American medical journals.

Even worse, mineral oil is indigestible. If taken with a meal, it surrounds food particles and makes them non-digestible. Vitamins that become clogged by mineral oil are evacuated without giving their value to your body.

Bran

To relieve constipation, one food which can help is bran. The milling industry first convinced farmers that it was good for horses. Next, the flour salesman told the public that bran had laxative properties.

But bran has this disadvantage: If its coarse grains start clumping together in the intestinal tract, they can irritate the digestive pathway. Whenever this occurs, it loses favor as a food supplement.

Cultured Milk

An effective cultured product is Acidophilous. The Bulgarian people still use this drink, which is rich in cultured bacteria. Buttermilk is another form of laxative favored by many. Buttermilk is acceptable, but there are better ways for the modern-day arthritic.

Psyllium Seeds

When soaked in water, psyllium seeds swell to twice their normal size—supposedly to clear the intestinal tract. The trick is to drink water before and after taking the seeds. In this manner you cause the seeds to exude a lubricating jelly which, reportedly, makes passage smoother. Frequently, however, psyllium seeds have been found to lodge in the intestinal walls and become foreign irritants.

Cascara Sagrada

A well-known laxative and stimulant, cascara sagrada is made from a shrub found in the western states. An American habit, hundreds of thousands use this type of product. It can give help. But cascara sagrada is not always tolerated by your system, and places added strain on the liver.

Milk of Magnesia

Popular in the United States, milk of magnesia is known as a mild purgative. Sooner or later almost every constipated arthritic tries it. With this product not too much damage is done to bodily oils.

Calomel

A white, tasteless, insoluble powder, calomel is capable of purging the body. But it, too, causes added work for liver.

Senna

The purgative known as senna is employed frequently in constipation among children and pregnant women. Senna—along with a drug called phenolphthalein—creates more havoc for the congested liver.

In addition, while carrying out waste, these laxatives may take with them some valuable digestive juices and food elements. They may remove the good, as well as the bad.

Agar-Agar

The Japanese think they have come up with a possible panacea for intestinal sluggishness in agar-agar. It's a seaweed found off the coast of Japan.

By absorbing and holding moisture, agar-agar prevents undue drying of the fecal mass. At the same time, however, it is non-digestible. Bulk results, which creates non-digestible and irritating materials. When non-digestible foreign particles from agar-agar envelop food particles with a film, the products for nutrition are not absorbed. Instead, they are excreted. Therefore, agar-agar is just as bad as mineral oil. In America, rhubarb and castor oil would be far better choices.

Colonic Irrigations and Enemas

The liquid methods—like colonic irrigations and enemas—we believe should be limited to use in post-operative cases, in hospitals and just for the chronically ill.

The previous paragraphs have presented a few of the ways by which we Americans try to solve our constipation problem. For the most part, we choose them because they are the easiest means to quick relief. If they fail to help us, and congestion remains a problem in the body, hemorrhoids may result.

Constipation is the most prevalent of human ailments. The arthritic has more than his share of this condition, so he must face the problem squarely. Try to do so, without trying to use water as the main measure.

How Much Water?

If the arthritic turns to drinking a great deal of water all day long, he will soon be surprised to find that water does NOT have the vital substance necessary to keep him regular. Almost everyone, with or without arthritis, makes this mistake. Extra water does not soften the mass in the colon which has become stagnant. The liver acts as a control—it inhibits extra water from reaching the colon as well as the bloodstream. At first, extra water will seem beneficial . . . but not for long.

The Pro and Con on Prune Juice

When an arthritic turns to prune juice, he is taking in concentrated fruit sugar. For a time, he will be helped. Soon however, its stimulative effect wears off. And "liquid" fruit sugar, of course, damages the oils trying to circulate within an arthritic.

Instead of drinking prune juice, eat prunes with breakfast several times a week. Or substitute black, unsulphured figs. Pressure-cook the prunes briefly. Prunes and figs will prove beneficial to combat constipation . . . and will do no harm to the bodily oils.

The Breakfast To Aid Regularity

Most constipated arthritics too often think of breakfast in terms of "bacon, eggs, toast, and coffee." Bacon and eggs do not add any stimulative effect to the colon. Toast and coffee contribute a mere trickle.

Many people swear by coffee as a laxative. Taken by itself, it may prove of some help. But, drink it 10 to 30 minutes before a meal or at least three hours after eating.

In this book, we have set up a better type of breakfast for arthritics. Consisting of buttered whole wheat toast, eggs, and a glass of room-temperature milk, eaten in that order. This gives the stomach the potential semi-solid mass. The whole wheat toast contributes the stimulating factor. A few leaves of green lettuce, with the morning meal, contain enough fiber to incite some more intestinal action.

Lettuce is optional, of course. It may sound strange as a breakfast food, but it does contain the right ingredients. Since no one wishes diarrhea or three bowel movements a day, we do not need any vegetable in the morning stronger than lettuce.

The fire—the burning of food—is now started. If you must drink anything between breakfast and lunch, make sure it is at least three hours after the first meal. And keep the liquid at room temperature or warm.

Lunch with the Right Ingredients

Lunch should also contain a stimulating factor which will aid the contraction and relaxation of the digestive tract muscles.

A lunch consisting of a grilled cheese sandwich should include a raw fruit or vegetable—so that the residue from the second meal will keep the mass moving. Celery, cucumber, or any laxative type vegetable is recommended. A portion of stewed prunes or raw, unsulphured (black) figs is gently laxative.

The correct type of lunch is outlined in Chapter XI. More varied lunches are included in Chapter XV, with the menus.

Afternoon Break

It is a long stretch between noon and six or seven o'clock when the third and often largest meal of the day is served. No one is expected to go without some liquid or solid food during this long interval. But try to avoid eating if you can, especially if you are unduly constipated and your body needs oils.

If necessary, drink water at room temperature. Providing it is at least three hours after lunch, or at least 10 minutes before dinner. Especially avoid iced water after a meal. Or you will congeal the oils still in the stomach and digestive tract . . . you will smother the food-burning fire which you set going at meal-time.

Any mid-afternoon snack or sandwich should contain a little butter or lettuce. Butter serves as a lubricant, and lettuce as a stimulant to food already ingested. Mayonnaise should not replace butter, because it will yield energy, not lubricants.

Dinner for Health and Enjoyment

At dinner time still remember the stimulating factor. Follow the dictates of taste and the needs of the bowel. The soup is beneficial, with its oils. The steak is delicious, and it can be improved by adding garlic. Garlic has a kick of its own, a stimulation for sluggishness.

For complete dinner menus, see Chapter XV. The meals were designed to aid arthritics, and the list of foods was made keeping constipation in mind.

The Great Danger

When arthritics get themselves constipated, not only do they fail to eat enough of the right foods, but they tend to go on liquid diets. That's the greatest danger. Because liquids can disqualify whatever good food they may have eaten.

If, in addition, people with constipation choose lemon juice and water, they will soon find that their skin, scalp, hair, ears, and nails are gradually drying out. Their gum lines may even start to recede. Lemon may help a rare few people with arthritis, but in the majority of cases it does harm.

Haste Makes Waste

The fast ways to regularity are not always the best. If constipation is present at the time of an appendicitis attack, harsh laxatives can lead to serious complications. The reports about burst appendices in the bodies of constipated people are not myths. All too many patients with colon discomfort have also found themselves with a ruptured appendix. The manufacturers of cathartics concede this fact, and mark appropriate warnings on the labels of their wares.

Analyze Your Problem

Arthritics who suddenly find themselves constipated should analyze the possible cause of their new misfortune. Here's how. . . .

The purpose of eating is to give cells and tissue their nourishment. This nourishment can only evolve when the food is broken down by digestive juices. The better one chews his food, the easier the work for the digestive juices.

Inside our bodies, chemical decomposition breaks down our food into tiny particles. From all this action, priceless vitamins, amino acids, sugar, salt, minerals—and microscopic oil by-products—are released by the small intestine into our bodies, for the purpose of nourishment, repair and storage.

Water in food, or milk or soup, accompanies foods as they pass through the digestive processes. The water adds solubility to the mixture, and makes the digestive task easier. Chewing your foods will permit easier digestion—because foods will then go into solutions of semi-liquids more readily.

We cannot emphasize too strongly or repeat too often this single fact. . . .

Let your foods be broken down and digested completely before you add any oil-free liquids.

Certain Foods Which Help

Arthritics should know how certain foods give bulk to the bracket-shaped large intestine. It has been scientifically proven that bulk can come from fruits and vegetables in the form of tough fibers. As competent as our digestive juices are, they cannot pulverize the indigestible fibers of fruits and vegetables. It is the skins of fruits, and the cellulose of vegetables, which remain as bulky residue.

Meat also yields tough fibers necessary for bulk. But avoid gorging yourself on meat, however. Eat larger portions of vegetables—like green celery, green lettuce, cucumber, raw carrots. And after lunch and dinner, eat whole raw fruits. (The fruits described on page 150 are best for arthritics.)

All the favorable talk about raw fruits and vegetables over the centuries is well founded. They do yield bulk, to aid regularity. For this purpose, do make them a habit.

On the other hand, don't believe claims that cake and candy will provide bulk for the constipated person. It's just not so. Keep your "sweet tooth" in check.

The Role of Bacteria

In the colons of constipated arthritics—in fact, in the bodies of everyone—exist millions and millions of intestinal bacteria. These bacteria are not like the bacteria of pneumonia, typhoid, and other germ-borne diseases. In the small intestine these "good" bacteria do a fine job. To make it possible for us to eat our required amounts of meat, these bacteria help disintegrate the unused particles of meat in our intestines.

Derivatives from protein, carbohydrates, oils, vitamins and minerals go into circulation, but the remaining wastes find their way into the large colon. The meats we eat leave a higher proportion of waste materials in our system than other types of food. Which means that the bacteria must spend a good deal of their time decaying meat particles.

Fresh Air as a Stimulant

Bacteria, hard at work in our system, need oxygen to fan the fire of digestion. Sizable quantities of fresh air can be of major aid to keep us regular.

Just spend a few minutes doing some deep inhaling—deep breathing in the morning when you arise. Again at night even while in bed, deep breathing exercises will help the 750,000,000 air cells in your lungs. The added air will awaken sluggish capillaries. Cause them to bring in oxygen and purify the wastes of the body.

Bulk foods during decomposition—if they are accelerated by helpful oxygen—have less chance of putrefaction.

In addition to aiding regularity, deep breathing will massage the lungs, heart, stomach, liver and spleen.

Recognize the Types and Symptoms of Constipation

Before you set out to gain more fresh air or try other methods of relief, it would be wise to know which type of constipation you have. There are three forms of this malady which can complicate arthritis:

Insufficient expressing of the excrement.
Insufficient quantity.
Evacuations of abnormally dry and hard stools.

The best way to check on your degree of constipation is to examine daily stools.

Continued evacuation of abnormally colored stools should cause an arthritic to consult his doctor. Lienteric stools containing much undigested food usually signify profound intestinal disorder.

If an arthritic discharges watery or serous stools, it may be due to nervousness, enteritis, or cholera. Pus-like stools may arise from ulceration along the digestive tract or from the rupture of an adjacent abscess in the bowel.

Lastly, arthritics should know that black, red, or bloody stools are danger signals. They are caused by internal hemorrhages, hemorrhoids, or by the use of drugs. Any of the above signs should cause you to seek medical attention promptly.

Other symptoms of constipation include fatigue, coated tongue, headaches, instability, nervousness, and bad breath.

Halitosis often results from excessive putrefaction in the colon. Sharp odors begin to arise in the colon and the air cells in the lungs begin to expel the toxic aromas. Decaying processes caused by over-indulgence in cake and candy lead to unfavorable changes in the breath. Free use of citric juices and soda pop can raise havoc with the digestive tract itself and cause it to degenerate. This also results in foul breath.

Skin blemishes can be evidence of constipation. They appear when toxic materials have become stagnant in your body.

Why are we devoting so much space to this problem of keeping regular? Because both arthritis and constipation can be caused by the same mistakes. And either ailment can be caused by the other.

Therefore, let us continue our examination into this vital subject.

A Leading Doctor's Opinion

The greatest work we have ever read in regard to constipation is a report in the *Journal of Laboratory and Clinical Medicine* by Dr. A. A. Fletcher of Toronto, Canada.

Dr. Fletcher mentions the experiments of Dr. R. McCarrison on sluggish monkeys. McCarrison reported that when he put monkeys on a bacteria free diet, high in starches, their colon lost muscle tone and the membrane degenerated. The bowel changes in his experimental animals were structurally and causally of the same nature as those found in human victims of chronically constipated arthritis.

Because the diets were sterilized, bacteria as a cause of arthritis was ruled out. These tests also condemned high starch intake in constipation. It was important to rule out bacteria, because until then rheumatologists were bacteria conscious. They thought that arthritis was caused by infection.

Dr. Fletcher also reported that when Dr. R. Pemberton restricted "inferior-type" starches in the diets (like cake and candy) of his human arthritic patients, their bowel actions were better, especially if vitamins were added to the diet. The doctors felt that a high starch diet precipitated borderline vitamin deficiencies. And that during the state of malnutrition, the body was more susceptible to germ invasion.

Dr. Fletcher's findings made it clear that more than one vitamin is deficient in the constipated person. Any diet which brings on constipation shows a multiple vitamin deficiency. The doctor stated, however, that it is predominantly a vitamin B deficiency which causes the bowel to break down and to lose its digestive action.

"Raw" Wheat Germ Experiments

To correct the constipation of his arthritic patients, Dr. Fletcher turned to raw wheat germ. He also tried wheat germ extracts and various forms of yeast. It was found that wheat germ is the most effective food to bring about improvement in the colon.

Dr. Fletcher wrote one more fact into his report which is the most significant of all. He stressed that, in addition to raw wheat germ, arthritics need a highly protective type diet. He said foods like meat, fish, fowl, eggs, liver, and milk must be consumed frequently.

(Does this sound familiar? Such a diet is exactly what we have been recommending for you throughout this book. Dr. Fletcher, whose report is Volume No. 15 dated back in 1929–30, was already practicing correct arthritic treatments.)

We, in turn, have developed additional methods to eat those foods in their proper order—so that you will obtain even greater amounts of vitamins and oils and gain relief even faster.

Summary of Best Aids

An entire picture of constipation has now been presented, and you have read the findings of leading medical authorities. The time has come to offer a solution which will bring you regularity.

For arthritics, we recommend the following measures and devices as the best:

"RAW" WHEAT GERM should be taken frequently. It is usually available in package, bottle or canned form at most grocery or health food stores. We suggest that you use two tablespoons of raw wheat germ on your breakfast cereal, or sprinkled on soup later in the day. Use it faithfully, for months if necessary.

For those with colitis, who cannot tolerate wheat germ, then wheat germ flake cereal served with milk may be substituted. Served with a few prunes or figs, wheat germ flake cereal is an EX-CELLENT laxative-type cereal to help improve regularity. Wheat germ flake cereal is a good source of the much needed Vitamin B. And more important—it is in natural food-form.

Raw wheat germ used sparingly (2 to 3 times a week) will do wonders for the human system in a period of 6 to 12 months.

ONIONS are the finest possible vegetable to relieve constipation. Use them in salads, on sandwiches, whenever you can.

Onion consumption can be planned to avoid the social error of bad breath. At the end of the day, when you are through with outside contacts, have a slice in a sandwich. If you put onion into your salads at lunch, the odor is soon dissipated. Once you have toned up your digestive tract, you can eat onions as seldom as two meals per week and you will still retain their beneficial stimulating factor.

GREEN CELERY, green lettuce, scallions, garlic and cucumbers are also bowel-muscle toning foods.

CARDINAL RULES TO REMEMBER
ABOUT CONSTIPATION

1. No white sugar—no sweets—no refined foods. White sugar, sweets and refined foods cause a gradual Vitamin B deficiency over the years. This deficiency leads to intestinal mucosa degeneration and loss of bowel muscle tone.
2. Add 1 to 2 tablespoonfuls of "raw" wheat germ to oatmeal (when served) or to some cereal or soup—2 to 3 times a week. This "raw" wheat germ gives back to the body a natural source of Vitamin B. This will help correct bowel-muscle tone gradually. If preferred, eat wheat germ flake cereal served with milk and prunes or figs several mornings a week. (Available at grocery or health food stores.)
3. Chew each mouthful of food extremely well . . . important.
4. Drink 1 to 2 glasses of "warm" water one hour before breakfast. If this isn't effective then take cold tap water one week and contrasting warm water on alternate weeks. (If cod liver oil is taken 1 to 2 hours before breakfast instead of before retiring, then drink your water about one-half hour before taking cod liver oil . . . or drink water for the day one hour "before" evening meal.)
5. Lean more to raw vegetables and fruits for bulk. If ulcer or colitis prevent this, cook these foods "slightly" in a pressure cooker.

6. Eat a few pressure-cooked prunes or raw, unsulphured (black) figs with breakfast meal. Pressure-cook briefly.
7. You may use a temporary laxative of your choice while bowel habits improve.

As a final suggestion to help constipated arthritics, we are printing (below) a special formula to encourage regularity. The following mixture has been used successfully in major hospitals.

FORMULA TO RELIEVE CONSTIPATION

¾ ounce powdered senna leaves
¼ ounce powdered slippery elm bark
½ ounce powdered charcoal
¾ ounce olive oil
¼ ounce glycerin
   (These products may be obtained in most drugstores.)
¾ pound black figs (not washed with sulphur)
⅜ pound raisins

The raisins and figs are run through a food chopper and pulverized.
Overlay all the other ingredients over the raisins and figs. Mix thoroughly.
Roll into about 10 walnut-shaped balls.
Use one every day, preferably before breakfast, until they work. Half or quarter portions may be used.

The above formula should bring you fast relief, which might cause the question to arise as to how much and how often you really need to "go."

Generally, one bowel movement a day is normal. Skipping a day is not anything to become alarmed about. In fact for some people a bowel movement every other day is considered adequate.

In conclusion, we have one point to emphasize. The formula and special laxatives which were given in this chapter will accomplish temporary aid. Then, for permanent regularity, an arthritic must depend on correct diet.

Chapter XX

Cortisone Can Help, But Not Cure

In the chapter you have just read we discussed many drugs and commercial laxatives which supposedly relieve constipation. Now, what about drugs to cure arthritis? Should we believe all the publicity about cortisone or the other "wonder drugs" for arthritics?

The next few pages will tell you what cortisone is, where it comes from, and the unvarnished truth about whether it will work.

Actually, cortisone is merely a hormone . . . one of 28 secreted by the adrenal glands right inside your body.

What is a hormone?

It is a substance which is manufactured in some bodily organ and is then transported to some other part of the body to produce a "strengthening" effect.

At birth, we are all given the ability to make our own cortisone. This is also true of the hormone known as insulin. Because our body makes natural insulin, most of us escape becoming diabetic. Another type, "sex hormones," make it possible for us to reproduce.

Cortisone Provided by Nature

Under favorable circumstances of correct diet, our adrenal glands can create very small quantities of cortisone every day. Without this minute supply, everyone would be an arthritic. We all must have this hormone, but victims of arthritis require a certain type of cortisone which has heavier consistency. Why?

Arthritics need a special "heavier" cortisone containing a "sticky quality." (This kind of cortisone can be obtained only by adding vitamin D oil to our daily diet.) What does the "stickiness" accomplish for our joints? It holds the lubricating oils in place and prevents them from seeping away from the joints.

A similar action is believed to take place in our connective tissues which surround our joints, as well as in the joint linings that we have been discussing.

Connective tissues contain collagen, a gluelike substance. Cortisone may increase the consistency of collagen—add an even greater "sticky quality." In other words, cortisone will help hold oils in their proper place throughout this whole general area. The very area where an arthritic needs oil most.

Many medical experts now agree on the use of

cortisone. Dr. R. H. Freyberg, a specialist at New York Hospital in Manhattan, believes that cortisone may have a working relationship with those tissues of our body known as "connective tissues."

The present popularity of cortisone to combat arthritis is due to Dr. Freyberg and other outstanding rheumatologists throughout the United States. They have been champions of this drug, and have conducted extensive research to prove its effectiveness. The widespread use of cortisone today is a tribute to their initiative, when we stop to think that it was introduced to the medical world only a very few years ago.

The Discovery of Cortisone

It all started at the Mayo Clinic as recently as 1949. In that year, Dr. P. Hench and Dr. E. Kendall—with their associates Dr. C. Slocumb and Dr. H. Polley—startled the entire field of medicine with their discoveries on the uses of "man-made" cortisone.

When the announcement of their important findings was made, I immediately boarded a plane and flew out to the Mayo Clinic in Rochester, Minnesota. I could not imagine or believe that a synthetic substance could perform "miracles" for arthritic bodies.

By making this trip to Minnesota, I was present at the Seventh International Congress on Rheumatic Diseases held at the Mayo Foundation. After hearing testimony on cortisone, I still did not believe that this drug was the complete answer to arthritis. It is not a permanent cure, and the past few years have proven I was right.

It is true that in certain kinds of arthritis, cortisone can turn off the pain within hours. But the relief is often temporary. Another advantage of taking cortisone is the fact that some chronic rheumatoid arthritics were then able to do exercises. By using their muscles, they were able to prevent wasting away and minimize crippling. Again, this gain was frequently nullified by relapses.

Cortisone, taken orally or by injection, does have an anti-inflammatory effect. For some rheumatoid arthritics it does lessen their joint stiffness, heat and swelling. But reports now indicate that some 85% of the cases later suffer relapses. And cortisone manufactured commercially has little or no effect whatsoever on osteo arthritis.

Any person or any chemical bringing even temporary relief deserves our thanks. Congratulations are in order to the doctors who developed cortisone and its uses. The only unfortunate fact is that cortisone does not bring lasting recovery.

And, we must add a definite warning that taking cortisone by prescription can cause a number of harmful reactions throughout your body. It may help arthritis, but irritate other tissues and organs.

The Disadvantages of Test-Tube Cortisone

Excessive use of cortisone, taken orally or by injection, can lead to many body disturbances. For example, it can affect menopause.

A large segment of arthritics are women in the forty- to fifty-year-old bracket. When they are in the menopausal stage, they must be doubly careful in using synthetic cortisone. Because the drug can cause accentuated flushing and high blood pressure.

Men and women of any age being treated with cortisone must be particularly careful to avoid falls or accidents, because of the great danger of breaking bones. Synthetic cortisone has a withdrawing effect on calcium and phosphorus and tends to leave bones in a brittle condition.

Cortisone has become so popular—yet is still so potentially dangerous if used excessively—we are going to print the following chart for your protection. Before you rush quantities of cortisone drugs into your system, read this list of dangers.

POSSIBLE COMPLICATIONS FROM THE EXCESSIVE USE OF CORTISONE

Too much cortisone can cause the following bodily conditions:
1. Increased swelling of hands, legs, etc., due to electrolyte imbalance.
2. Cause carbohydrate imbalance, leading to diabetes.
3. Ballooning of the face, make you "moon faced."

4. Growth of hair in the wrong places (causing mustaches on women, etc.).
5. Creates acne, skin blemishes.
6. May add excessive weight, make you obese.
7. Cause mental depression, nervousness, moodiness.
8. Elevate your blood pressure.
9. Lead to blood clotting disturbances.
10. Bring on abnormally fast heart beat.
11. Start hemorrhages of the gastro-intestinal tract.
12. Menstruation can be decreased, delayed, or completely eliminated.
13. Softening of the bones; danger of fractures.
14. Reactivates peptic ulcers.
15. Can develop larger tonsils.
16. Slows down your adrenal glands.
17. Reduces the action of your thyroid gland.
18. Can lead to insomnia.

For the reasons shown above, we now know that we do not want large quantities of cortisone poured into our bodies. In arthritis, it is the quality of the cortisone which counts.

What, then, can improve the cortisone? What, in our bloodstream, can stimulate the adrenal glands into producing a higher quality natural cortisone?

We know that cortisone is secreted from the outer bark or layers of the adrenals. We also know that it takes steroid substances to activate these glands.

Vitamin D is a steroid substance. The only kind of vitamin D which can do the stimulating job is found in cod liver oil. (Milk, eggs, and butter are foods which can also contribute a trickle of this vitamin D activating substance. But only if the food is prepared properly and consumed in the correct order—as listed in the menus of Chapter XV.)

The Whole Answer in Plain Words

We maintain that an arthritic who takes his cod liver oil correctly (described in Chapter XVII) can make his own cortisone. By emulsifying his cod liver oil with orange juice, he can send oil bubbles containing steroid vitamin D to his adrenal glands . . . stimulate the glands into producing higher quality natural cortisone.

Without this better grade of hormone in your connective tissue, your tissue fluids gel and stiffen instead of functioning normally. And why is the quality of your cortisone not up to par? Because, for all these years, <u>the stimulative effect of vitamin D and iodized oil has been missing from your blood-stream!</u>

Final Conclusions About "Wonder Drugs"

Before ending this chapter about cortisone, here are a few words to the wise about two other commercially manufactured products.

You may have heard a good deal about ACTH. It deserves some consideration. ACTH is another hormone which can benefit only those with rheumatoid arthritis. Again, victims of osteo arthritis are forgotten. ACTH is made from the pituitary gland. It can temporarily stimulate the adrenal glands into producing more cortisone.

Dr. E. F. Rosenberg of the Michael Reese Hospital in Chicago skillfully sums up the action of ACTH on the adrenal glands. He believes that ACTH causes cortisone to be produced through its stimulus of the adrenal enzymes, using ascorbic acid and cholesterol as raw materials. (Dr. Rosenberg's report on ACTH forms a section of Comroe's book on arthritis.)

In the cod liver oil and orange juice mixture we have a parallel. Orange juice contains ascorbic acid. The oil globule, a sterol, takes on an adhering film of ascorbic acid. When the two, as a unit, reach the adrenal glands, they can stimulate the glands into making better-grade cortisone.

HYDROCORTISONE is still another drug being prescribed these days for arthritics. When injected directly into the joint, it has been found capable of anti-inflammatory effect. Temporary effect.

Pioneering in this field is Dr. J. L. Hollander of Philadelphia. He recently edited a valuable book, *Comroe's Arthritis and Allied Conditions* (published in 1953 by Lea and Febiger).

Dr. Hollander believes that these injections of hydrocortisone serve as a lubricating oil to the joint, by diffusing the ingredients of the hormone into the cells of joint linings.

Be it the use of cortisone, hydrocortisone, ACTH, or any other drug, medical records are now proving that they are all temporary aids. For lasting results, we will have to depend on our own adrenal glands and their ability to make better-grade natural cortisone.

Taking drugs can become a habit or a fad. Almost to the point of just trying to do "something" so you can say you're fighting your arthritis.

Some people even turn to superstition. For an interesting, sometimes humorous, and helpful

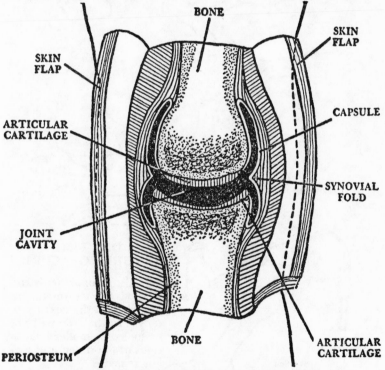

A TYPICAL JOINT—Where Arthritis Strikes

chapter on superstitions about arthritis, the next part of this book will take you back through the centuries. . . .

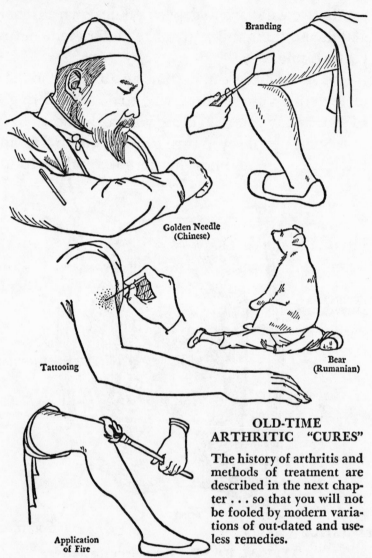

Branding

Golden Needle
(Chinese)

Tattooing

Bear
(Rumanian)

Application
of Fire

OLD-TIME ARTHRITIC "CURES"

The history of arthritis and methods of treatment are described in the next chapter . . . so that you will not be fooled by modern variations of out-dated and useless remedies.

Chapter XXI

Superstitions and False Remedies

If we are to find a modern cure for arthritis, we must first know all the past methods which have failed. We must eliminate all of the wrong theories, learn to disregard just plain superstitions.

Any scientist—when he sets out to discover the correct medicine or treatment—will first go back into history to consult centuries of past knowledge. He will want to know what other scientists did wrong, and why these mistakes were made.

You, too, should be interested in knowing the false remedies, the quack ideas and the failures of old-time medicine men. Unless you know the difference between a "legend" and a correct cure, how can you hope to choose the right road to recovery?

So, this chapter will trace the course of medical progress back through hundreds of years. By reading about these superstitions and strange treatments, you will be able to see how arthritic research has grown. You will be able to recognize the wisdom —or the false hope—offered to modern patients.

Many of the methods used today to fight arthritis began ages ago. Some brilliant men and women, the best brains of their day, were interested in arthritis. Read on, and learn what they contributed toward helping you.

First, let's look at the black side of the picture. The terrifying treatments and painful mistakes which were tried on arthritics throughout the world. . . .

Acupuncture

The ancient Chinese—to fight arthritis—pricked the skin with needles made from different kinds of metals. When the surface puncture did not bring relief, they turned to acupuncture—piercing the deeper-lying organic structures.

The purpose of this "medical stunt" is still debatable. Although it was believed that piercing altered nerve currents and blood vessel reflexes. Another drastic form of "cure" was burning with fire-soaked fibres. Small cones of fibres—taken from a flax-like plant called artemisia—were drenched with saltpeter, placed in the inflamed region of the body, and lighted! Think of the excruciating pain . . . and be glad you live in modern times.

These terrible customs were not limited to the Chinese. The Japanese, Tibetans, and Malayans also employed the same tactics.

Tattooing

The highly decorated bodies of the African Negro are considered beautiful among their fellows. But did you know that a tattoo was also supposed to ease their arthritic pains? Certain types of tattooing have long been used to chase evil spirits. It hasn't worked yet. In fact, I actually met a tattooed man in a circus side show who has arthritis!

Hindu Habits Hurt

About 1000 B.C. the Hindus of India became convinced that superficial arthritis was a skin and muscle disturbance, and they thought that nerve and joint conditions were deeper organic malfunctions. To cure it was a question of alteration or elimination.

So, the Hindus turned to vegetable drugs to cleanse their bodies. Their methods of counterirritation included liniments, applying blood-sucking leeches to the body, bleeding of veins and cauterization by burning. They even tried cutting . . . making small superficial incisions which they termed scarification. The result: Soon they had scars and arthritis!

Hippocrates

Hippocrates, the immortal Greek, contributed a great deal to medicine. But he was just as wrong as everyone else about arthritis. He believed, way back there around the year 450 B.C., that arth

216 SUPERSTITIONS AND FALSE REMEDIES

ritics should be "drained." He insisted that in-
flammatory fluids should be drained through the
skin. Today, it is known that all too many cases of
this illness do not show any sign of fluid.

Hippocrates also thought of arthritis in terms
of retained body poisons—especially in the female
sex, when scanty menstruation or menopause was
present. The Greek scholar criticized the men, and
blamed their arthritis on excessive wine and sexual
relations. (Hippocrates was wrong! Sex habits are
not related in any way with arthritis.)

Wine

On the matter of excessive wine drinking,
however, he was on the right track. The fact that
the value of oils can be largely destroyed by wines
is a correct observation. Consuming wine—in great
quantity, like the Greeks of old—would take a
drastic toll of ingested fats.

The heavy wine-drinking in those days had an
injurious effect on metabolism. Kept the liver in a
constant state of repairing itself. No wonder thousands of people in those days became victims of
gouty arthritis.

Purging the Body

According to Hippocrates, pain above the diaphragm could be eliminated by forced vomiting.

And, he said, all other pain below the waist could be removed by downward purging—by the use of strong laxatives or enemas.

Can you possibly imagine an enema relieving the pain in a finger of the left hand? According to physicians of old, why not? The finger is below the diaphragm—and a warm saline solution can cleanse the blood. From the standpoint of logic, Hippocrates went too far with his ideas about purging. In all probability he urged sweating and bleeding, too.

The Greeks Blamed Uric Acid and Horseback Riding

In early Greece, too much Spartan horseback riding was considered a cause for arthritis. If they had a painful hip, it was supposedly due to riding —or deposits of uric acid in the hip joints.

Grecians thought that the sciatic nerve was accumulating sticky deposits of black bile. Horseback riding might—through constant friction—injure a susceptible joint inclined to accumulate uric acid.

Now, more than 2,000 years later, the term uric acid has replaced the title of black bile. Acids and friction do complicate arthritis, so there was a germ of truth in those early Greek ideas.

Turning the Heat on Arthritis

There must be millions of arthritics throughout the United States who have arthritis of the spine. Fortunately for them, the practices of Hippocrates are outmoded. His theory of cure for this malady consisted of cauterization . . . by burning!

The back, on both sides of the spinal column, were given four burns. Then, 15 more burns were inflicted on each side of the spine. And, to top it off, two burns were added to each side of the neck. There are not many persons, arthritic or otherwise, who could endure this form of torture. (Personally, we would probably rather have arthritis!)

Take Your Choice . . .

During the first, second and sixth centuries A.D. Largus, Galen, and Alexander Trallianus led the battle against arthritis.

All three of these Roman doctors thought of the disease as an alteration and elimination problem. Largus' method was to prescribe complicated herbal mixtures. Wine with wool fat. Fennel and flax-seed. Blends of vinegar and active lime.

This old-time expert recommended vomiting high on his list of cures. Largus would bring in a patient, and he would cause vomiting by tickling the throat with peacock feathers. If arthritis could be cured by the use of peacock feathers, those birds would indeed be popular today.

Galen's favorite counter-irritant for fused

arthritis was to apply a mixture of sharp cheese and a salted pork solution directly to the diseased joint.

Alexander Trallianus, the third great physician of the trio, had a few ideas of his own about arthritis. For bile disturbances he prescribed cooling and soothing remedies. For phlegm, he recommended stimulants. But for practically everything he prescribed, Trallianus was guided by astronomy!

This medicine man Trallianus was a stargazer. He believed that people were influenced by climatic conditions and signs. (Office hours on clear nights only . . . otherwise, the beclouded doctor is out.)

Ignipuncture

The Chinese in olden times relied on acupuncture. The Arabians had their own methods, which centered on ignipuncture. (Meaning they cauterized by hot irons!)

Depending on the site, size, and form of the arthritis, they applied different types of hot irons. They seared through the entire skin as deeply and as near to the joint as could be humanly tolerated. This practice finally reached such a painful point that even the Arab surgeons didn't want any part of it.

So, it fell to Arab barbers and laymen to carry out the burning routine. Because of this quackery, ignipuncture fell into disrepute. It had been the habit to let the open burns remain unbandaged, to allow the diseased fluids to exude. Infections followed, and the arthritic soon had more trouble to cope with than before the treatment.

Since the Year 5000 B.C.

Yes, as far back as 5000 B.C. the Chinese had arthritis. So did the Japanese, Tibetans, Malayans, Hindus, and the early Greeks and Romans. I repeat, their excessive drinking of wines may have been one cause for the disease. Today, Americans drink less wine at their meals, but we have added copious amounts of fruit juices, tea, and parasitic carbonated water.

Now, as the carbonated beverage fad makes its way into foreign lands, watch the increase of oil deficiency diseases. Watch the growth of arthritis in Egypt, Greenland, and Alaska in the next ten years! Why? It could be the new soda-pop fans.

Paracelsus

During the first half of the sixteenth century there was still another immortal Roman physician. His name was Paracelsus. And he went to great lengths to make his fellow-practitioners believe that arthritis was curable.

First, Paracelsus traveled the length and breadth of Europe, asking everyone their opinion as to the cause and cure of arthritis. He questioned alchemists, the pharmacists of his day, lay healers, barber surgeons, shepherds, even gypsies—asking whether they obtained results with herbs and vegetable drugs. He also collected and studied all the knowledge of arthritis from practicing physicians of many different nations. So, when Paraclesus said that arthritis was curable, he was giving the combined opinion of his day.

An Early Expert, Close to the Truth

Paracelsus classified the many arthritics as victims of a tartaric disease. The word tartar originated from the Greek word for wine precipitation.

What irony! The great Paracelsus was calling arthritis a wine-like precipitate. He was very close to the correct answer . . . way back in the 16th Century! It may well have been excessive wine-intake—practiced in those days—which actually prevented oils from ever reaching their correct equilibrium and final nourishment of the joints. The wine was altering the oil composition of protein, carbohydrate, or simple oil products—robbing arthritic joints. Tartaric deposits pointed emphatically to the cause of pain. Today, in our research, we are following through where Paracelsus left off.

A Contribution from France

Another European physician, a Frenchman named Ambroise Paré, was also intensely interested in arthritis. And he shared some of the views of his contemporary Paracelsus.

Both believed that the body of an arthritic needed special help from the liver. Since they were of the yellow and black bile school, they felt that the liver must remain unobstructed, to prevent defects in the uric acid metabolism.

Ambroise Paré was perfectly right about the liver being important. (This book has a whole chapter on the subject, Chapter XVIII.) But on his next idea, Ambroise Paré was dead wrong.

Paré was of the opinion that color-complex is also responsible for arthritis. A dark-complexioned person, he said, was a born arthritic. That is ridiculous! Red-heads, blondes, or albinos have an equal chance of becoming arthritic. The bloodstreams and digestive juices in people with dark complexions work in precisely the same manner—in regard to fats and oils—as those of people with light coloring.

Hemorrhoidal Bleeding

In foreign countries, many centuries ago, hemorrhoidal bleeding was considered a cure. It was an attempt to rid the body of all noxious abdominal fluids.

Today if we were to induce hemorrhoids to prevent arthritis, it would be a useless crime.

They Did Their Best

Should we condemn all counter-irritation measures?

We know that counter-irritation does not improve the quality of the bloodstream from the point of view of blood chemistry. But ancient physicians did obtain relief from some diseases by ridding the body of its detrimental fluids. And, even today, an arthritic coming into a hospital is thoroughly checked for excessive red blood cells and hemoglobin—rather than for "fullness of blood" as the ancients called it.

Gold Salts

By reviewing these old-time treatments and superstitions, we have been trying to show how modern "cures" for arthritis actually were born centuries ago. When you have gone seeking relief, too often you have been told old ideas—dressed up in new language. Take the case of "Gold Salts" . . . which may have been prescribed to you as a "surefire answer" to your pains. . . .

"Gold Salts" were first tried on arthritics back in the 16th Century! Porterius, a French physician, first used colloidal gold compounds.

Chrysotherapy, as it is called, is regarded as an effective mode of therapy to stimulate lymphatic glands into withdrawing foreign materials from your system. We cannot affirm or deny the potential powers of gold metallic salts. But let's look at the record . . . here's the price you may have to pay. . . .

Using metallic gold salts has been known to cause inflammation of the skin, fever, stomatitis, neuritis, dizziness, albuminuria, white blood cell dyscrasia, or a deficiency of red blood cells. It seems hardly worth the effort to invite any of these afflictions in a doubtful attempt to rid oneself of arthritis.

The Golden Needle

We have been explaining chrysotherapy, so let's not omit the Chinese version of gold salt injection. The Chinese inject the gold in the form of a golden needle—which they leave sticking in the troubled area of the body for a painful length of time.

The magazine section of a New York newspaper published a photograph showing an elderly Chinese seated in passive resignation—with a large golden needle piercing through many layers of clothing into his arm. (This same magazine showed another superstition, displaying how powder made from the skin of snakes would supposedly cure rheumatism.)

Gold salts, golden needle or snake powder . . . they may all be just about equal in their lack of effectiveness.

Do Bacteria Cause Arthritis?

Purgation and counter-irritation received a great setback with the rise of bacteriology. Even gold salts were forgotten for a while.

Arthritis specialists all began looking for bacterial infections. Infected tonsils, appendices, teeth —all were taken out—until it was noticed that arthritic shoulders, knees, or inflamed joints still did not heal.

Removing an infected organ will not stop arthritis.

Bacteriology is not the answer to this disease. No germ carries it, or causes it. Arthritis is not contagious . . . we are convinced it is constitutional and an oil deficiency

Potatoes and Chestnuts

Believe it or not, some arthritics in America still practice the old custom of carrying around an old dried potato in their pocket. This supposedly fights off attacks of pain. Other people swear by chestnuts.

Bear Treatment

The above "charms" are almost as queer as the Rumanian "bear cure."

In Rumania, the gypsies place an arthritic patient flat on the ground. The poor human lies prone, while a large brown bear tramples up and down his spine. If the sufferer escapes a broken back, the numbness from having 300 pounds of bear on him dulls the other pains.

Copper and Zinc

When will people learn that arthritis is a lack of specific oils feeding the synovial linings of our joint cavities?

That's the only fact you need to remember. Instead, some people still wear a copper bracelet on their left ankle—or a zinc plate in the heel of their right shoe—and <u>hope</u> to cure arthritis by this "magic."

To the Spa, for Mineral Water

Perhaps you are a believer in spring water, or mineral water. They, too, are classified as laxatives and are called "good for arthritics." Many misled people afflicted with arthritis flock to the spas . .

in order to be near natural sources of mountain water.

My research indicates that the only relief they receive comes mainly from the relaxation. It's not the water, it's the rest and vacation. And, at a spa, perhaps the victims have a more balanced diet than they are accustomed to eating. Except for these benefits, the soothing powers of physiotherapy and hydrotherapy can be vastly over-rated.

Heat Applications

Also under the heading of physiotherapy come the superstitions of hot water bottles, rags dipped in kerosene, burnt feathers and red flannels. All these provide bodily warmth. So does sun bathing. But . . . the dangers of heat applications and too much sun bathing are great. For arthritics, the sun may "bleed out" the very oils you are trying to save in your bodily joints. Unless your diet is correct—and contains goodly supplies of the right oils—be careful how much sunning you do.

Temporary relief may be obtained by vitamin D synthesis and blood vessel dilation due to sun rays. But we're looking for a <u>permanent</u> recovery.

Oils Are the Answer

To counter-act the bleeding of oils by the sun is another reason you should use cod liver oil. More and more medical authorities are beginning to agree that cod liver oil is valuable.

Dr. Marie and Dr. Strümpell, and other famous 20th Century physicians, viewed cod liver oil as an ally in arthritis therapy. Instead of irritating and inflaming your organs, it has the power of synthesizing new, reparative tissue while lubricating the joint lining.

Use Your Mind, Not Magic

This chapter has reviewed many of the most common superstitions and misconceptions on how to cure arthritis. Some of the methods are so weird that they are humorous.

Let's not fool ourselves. There is no "magic formula" to defeat this disease. It will take intelligent thinking, common sense. Compare the recommendations in this book—the sound, safe dietary approach—with the wild schemes down through the centuries which you have just been reading about. Make your own choice.

Chapter XXII

The Rate of Recovery

As you have been reading this book, learning new facts about yourself and the foods which go into your body, one major question may have been growing in your mind. "If I avoid superstitions and false cures, and if I adopt the plan outlined in these pages . . . how long will it take me to get well?"

The answer as to <u>when</u> and how soon you will stop having arthritic pains can be given in one sentence: "It is entirely up to you." Will you be faithful and follow a proper diet, as well as taking the cod liver oil each night? If you insist on "cheating" some here and there, it will take a longer period to bring you relief.

Should you wish to splurge when you are dining out or attending a social function, for instance, leaving the diet one night in a month or so will do no harm. But you cannot constantly forego your routine, and expect to gain maximum benefits in a short time.

An avid coffee drinker will probably find it very difficult at first to give up his favorite beverage. Over-indulgence in rich food, sweets, pastries, and

229

desserts will retard recovery. To go on with such facts would only be repetition, so we shall sum it up by saying: "If you're going to follow this dietary plan, then follow it!"

Next, we come to the cod liver oil phase recommended in this book. Some of you may shudder at the idea of taking this most fishy tasting liquid. But we are seeking health, not delicacies to please our palates. And here's an interesting fact which we have not emphasized as yet . . . you may use mint flavored cod liver oil. Such a product has appeared in drugstores lately, and this mint-flavored variety has a much better taste. More important, it contains all the same benefits as regular cod liver oil.

Be faithful to your cod liver oil routine and you will shorten the span of your pain-ridden days.

Where you have had days, months, even years of discomfort, you will suddenly realize that you are now having "good days" with no pain at all. The change itself is a gradual process. But your number of "good days" will keep increasing until you are no longer classified as an "arthritic."

Two other factors to be considered in your rate of recovery are the parts of the body in which you have arthritis, and the degree to which the disease has already progressed before you read this book.

Generally speaking, after taking cod liver oil daily, your fingers and your arms will lose their stiffness and swelling first. Arthritis of the back and spine will require the longest time before any change is noticed. The oil will be distributed to all other parts of the body before the painful spine will gain enough for relief.

Reports coming in to me by mail from hundreds of arthritics reveal that they show signs of "good days" in as little as one or two weeks. Even the more chronic cases take only six months to a year. In other words you should take the oil for two months or so, then look for external signs that your body has received lubrication . . . and keep the plan going until you have given it a fair trial. You may be surprised at how very early it works for you, even before two months.

Remember, occasionally, it is also possible that you may take the oil for two months and be feeling quite well, when all at once some pain may re-occur. This is not unusual and is no cause for alarm. This brief relapse has taken place in a number of cases immediately before the complete and final disappearance of pain.

To those with frozen or disfigured joints, there is nothing other than possible surgery which will alter your condition. However, our oil and dietary plan will prevent such cases from advancing any farther and will reduce your pain. This is a blessing in itself. But we are the first to admit and remind you that once nodes are formed and joints become

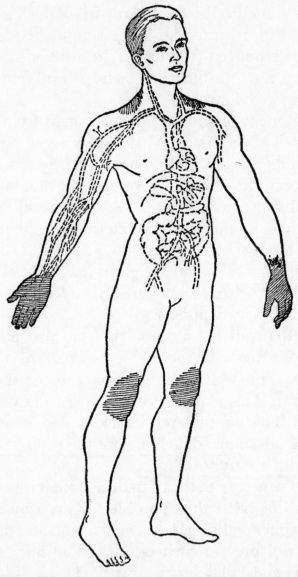

The distance which cod liver oil and other lubricating oils must travel—in order to reach your arthritic joints to reduce friction and ease pain and swelling, determines, in part, your rate of recovery. *Also, if the scalp, hair, ears, and outer skin of the body are dry, then added weeks of cod liver oil will be needed.*

fused, all the cod liver oil in the world will not return bones to their normal shape.

There has been a tendency for some deformed arthritics, and even some less serious cases, to continue taking cod liver oil for periods longer than six months. We repeat, you cannot change deformity that way. And anyone continuing with cod liver oil and orange juice for six months should then take a rest for two weeks or so. To avoid the remote chance of becoming temporarily allergic to the fruit sugar and citric acid in the orange juice.

For those chronic cases only—who have been on the regime for six months—and not for the millions of average arthritics—we recommend that you begin using cod liver oil by itself, once a week. Taken alone more of the oil will be trapped by the liver, but approximately 50% will still get through to your lymphatic system and to your joints. (For millions of arthritics we emphasize again that you should emulsify the oil and you should mix it with orange juice—to get much more than 50% of the oil past the liver! The above two paragraphs have been directed at only special cases of advanced arthritis.)

This chapter has told arthritics how long it will take them to become well. We know that we have been giving you the correct information, because we have seen with our own eyes hundreds of people who used our dietary plan successfully. We have seen arthritics who actually left wheelchairs and crutches behind them—to walk again because of these discoveries.

Each day brings more and more mail from grateful readers, telling of their quick recoveries. The fact is, I am grateful to them for having the confidence to follow my recommendations and for the way they have so faithfully followed the diets. I always appreciate receiving letters addressed to me in care of West Hartford, Connecticut, because each day the mailman brings to my home proof that my findings really work.

Most truthfully, I cannot claim to have "discovered" cod liver oil as an agent against arthritis. In fact, earlier in this book I have cited cases where leading doctors have used this oil for years. Perhaps what I have developed, after 14 years of research in the arthritic field, is the co-ordinating of a correct diet and a more effective and standard method of using the oil.

It is my hope that the knowledge you have gained in this book will help you as much as it has helped others.

Chapter XXIII

The Answer to Your Key Questions

Since writing the first edition of this book, four years ago, questions about diet have come to me from thousands of arthritics in all parts of the United States. Everyone has a slightly different problem, and the mail has been heavy with queries.

In addition, as some readers may know, I have been invited to lecture in many leading cities. To keep these speaking engagements—and to conduct on-the-spot research among arthritics—I have traveled six times across the United States. From Connecticut to California and back. Six coast-to-coast trips, with north and south journeys in between, covering more than 100,000 miles!

These travels have included stops at the foremost centers of arthritic research at hospitals, clinics and medical offices to talk with scores of doctors. We are still seeking knowledge, and we will continue to do so until arthritis can be conquered by modern science.

My findings have caused comment and interest in every city along the way. Physicians, laymen, readers . . . all have asked searching questions about my dietary approach. And, frequently, I hear

235

the same questions again and again. In this chapter I will repeat—and answer—the most popular questions, the ones I hear most often.

Perhaps the list of questions which follows shortly will serve to summarize in quick fashion some of the things you have been wondering about while you've been reading. They may be the questions you would ask, if we ever had the pleasure of meeting personally.

For that matter, it is quite possible that you and I may meet each other in the course of my travels. A few months from now, I may come to your city or home town to talk with arthritics. Or, if I have already visited your city, I may be back again. Because, quite often, the interest shown has brought me back to give a second or third lecture in the same auditorium.

Perhaps a relative or friend of yours has already attended one of my lectures. If so, they can give you added facts about arthritis, which they learned during my talks. So that you will know where I have been, and whether your city might expect me back, here is a list of the cities where I have addressed audiences on my recent lecture tour:

Philadelphia, Los Angeles, Detroit, San Francisco, Cleveland, Miami, Washington, D.C., Denver, Minneapolis, St. Paul, Houston, Cincinnati, Indianapolis, New Orleans, Buffalo, Pittsburgh,

Milwaukee, Memphis, Toledo, Columbus, Dayton, Rochester, Hartford, Louisville, Little Rock, Birmingham, Tulsa, Wichita, Lincoln, Hot Springs, Phoenix, Oakland, Sacramento, San Jose, Grand Rapids, Syracuse, Tampa, St. Petersburg, Orlando, Jacksonville, Worcester, New Bedford, Manchester, Atlantic City, Santa Monica, Allentown and San Antonio.

If your city is not included in the above group, it probably will be before too long. And I will be returning to many of the above localities to further my research among arthritics, Again, may I express my gratitude for the response and reception which has been given me everywhere. The audiences have come—in gatherings from 100 townsfolk to as many as 8,000 people at a single lecture—and they have listened, learned and then practiced my method.

All told, tens of thousands of Americans have met with me personally to discuss our mutual interest—arthritis. And, as I say, at the end of each lecture, thousands of them have stood up and asked me a dietary question. Here are your questions answered ... a resumé of the queries I hear most often.

1. Question. How many times a week should I eat eggs?
   Answer. An egg should be eaten at least every other day. Preferably more often. (Soft boiled eggs are best.)
2. Q. Can I drink milk other than at meal time during hot weather?

A. Because it contains oil, milk can be had at any time. (Drink it at room temperature.)

3. **Q.** Should whole wheat toast and butter be eaten first with breakfast, lunch and dinner?

   A. No. Although excellent . . . use variety. Soup or some solid food are good choices.

4. **Q.** How about frozen foods?

   A. Frozen fruits and vegetables are good to use frequently.

5. **Q.** Is it all right to eat salty crackers with soup?

   A. Salt is constipating to many arthritics. Use moderation.

6. **Q.** What cooked vegetables can be eaten?

   A. Most any cooked vegetable is acceptable, but try to lean toward raw vegetables.

7. **Q.** What kind of figs or prunes can be taken as a laxative?

   A. Unsulphured figs and good-grade organically-grown prunes are best choices.

8. **Q.** What solid foods should I be on guard against?

   A. Citric fruit, white bread, sweets, and highly spiced foods. No sour tomatoes or pickles.

9. **Q.** May I take the cod liver oil mixture in the morning, instead of just before going to bed?

   A. Yes, but at least 1 to 2 hours before breakfast, even if you have to delay your breakfast until later in the morning. However, the oil is still more effective taken at night.

10. **Q.** When should I eat raw fruit?

    A. Preferably at the end of your meal. Or, if you wish, two to three hours after mealtime

11. **Q.** Since certain fish tastes unpleasant to me, can I use canned tuna instead?

    A. Yes, but drain away and discard the cotton-seed or soya bean oil in the can. These oils are the wrong kind for arthritics.

12. **Q.** Can I substitute bran occasionally for oatmeal?

    A. Yes. Other cereals recommended are wheat cereals and whole grain types.

13. **Q.** Can wheat germ be eaten with oatmeal occasionally?

A. Yes. And raw wheat germ can even be used with soups or salads. Make sure it is "raw" wheat germ.

14. **Q.** Is salt alright to use?
A. Use salt sparingly.

15. **Q.** Can I eat watermelon or cantaloupe as dessert?
A. Minimize your eating of watermelon, because of its sugar and water. Cantaloupe, crenshaw and casaba melon are excellent as dessert dishes.

16. **Q.** Should I use gravies at mealtime?
A. Only natural gravies from broiled lean meats, or from butter used in broiling.

17. **Q.** What is a good raw, green vegetable?
A. Green celery and green lettuce are the best.

18. **Q.** What is a good "snack" sandwich?
A. Lettuce and tomato on whole wheat buttered toast. Or, a grilled whole wheat cheese sandwich.

19. **Q.** Is it true that arthritics are generally more thirsty than others?
A. People who have oil deficiencies (arthritics) frequently crave water. As the deficiency is corrected, your thirst will be stabilized.

20. **Q.** Can broiled liver and lean steaks take the place of liver and iron capsules?
A. No. Those foods give only small quantities of iron. Concentrated liver and iron capsules are a better way to reintroduce iron into your system.

21. **Q.** Is there any danger of my taking too much cod liver oil?
A. No. However, one tablespoon a day should be used as an average. Two tablespoons should be maximum.

22. **Q.** Can cod liver oil capsules be used in place of the pure cod liver oil?
A. No. Capsules merely serve as vitamin supplements. The pure liquid oil is needed as a lubricant.

23. **Q.** Must I eat three meals a day?
A. Yes, if humanly possible.

24.   Q. Can I drink a glass of milk as my whole breakfast?

A. If in a hurry, now and then. But the body needs more than milk to balance a breakfast. Certainly milk is a lot better than just a cup of black coffee.

25.   Q. How does saccharin compare to sugar in the arthritic diet?

A. If you feel you must have coffee, drink it at the right time, and the use of saccharin is recommended. Sugar is out—in all forms.

26.   Q. Will the dietary regime in this book help victims of bursitis, neuritis and gout?

A. Yes, these ailments will be alleviated by following the dietary plan in this book.

27.   Q. Can I use skim milk in my coffee?

A. Yes, as long as you drink the coffee at the specified time in relation to your entire meal. Do not drink skimmed milk with meals in any form.

28.   Q. If I take milk of magnesia or some laxative at night, can I still take the cod liver oil before going to bed?

A. Yes, take the laxative (any other but mineral oil) ½ hour to 1 hour before the cod liver oil and at least 2-3 hours after dinner. Mineral oil, if used, should be taken in the morning; if cod liver oil is used at night. As final choice —if you use mineral oil at night—use mineral oil only on alternate nights and skip the cod liver oil on that night.

29.   Q. I would like to try the cod liver oil, but can I start with smaller amounts?

A. Yes. If you wish—you may take a teaspoon of cod liver oil mixed thoroughly with 2 tablespoonsful of orange juice—every other night. Progress is slower—but at least you will be on the right track.

30.   Q. Since almost everyone gets arthritis sooner or later, wouldn't it be wise for everyone to take cod liver oil as a preventative measure?

A. Yes. If one automatically eats the right food and has correct eating habits . . . one tbsp. cod liver oil a month would be ample preventative amount. Above all, people should correct their eating habits.

Chapter XXIV

What the Future Holds for Arthritics

As we come to this, the final chapter of our book, one great question remains. Can a victim of arthritis expect a complete cure?

Phrased in another way . . . how close is medical science to finding the whole answer to this dread disease? Let us take stock, add up the discoveries, and look into your future.

What has the arthritic to look forward to? A great deal, we're happy to say.

More than ever before, efforts are being made to make the life of the arthritic more livable. For the first time in the history of mankind, the arthritic cripple is no longer a silent sufferer. Thanks to a pioneer named Dr. Philip S. Hench of the Mayo Clinic, arthritis is receiving public attention and is being studied thoroughly on a world-wide scale.

New research on the arthritic and his diet is starting in the United States Public Health Service Hospital in Bethesda, Maryland. These dietary tests may well bring us the solution of the problem.

Let us not forget that until a few years ago members of the American medical profession were still debating amongst themselves about arthritis.

Prior to the discovery of cortisone and similar compounds, there was not even a standard way to gain temporary relief from the disease. In more recent years, vitamin D drugs and gold salt injections at least stirred up controversies to create interest in the problem.

More Doctors Needed

Of the 180,000 doctors in the United States today, only about 20,000 to 30,000 seem willing to tackle arthritis or specialize in it. Of these, the internists insist that this disease is their problem. The orthopedic surgeons consider arthritis a part of their field. More physicians, trained in rheumatology, are needed on the American scene if we are going to move forward to even greater progress.

As a final summary, let us review current drugs and treatments to see the extent of our "progress" in modern times. Here's a check list for you on so-called "cures" which will not bring permanent relief for your arthritis. We'll start the resumé with something as well known as simple aspirin.

Aspirin Is No Cure

Just about all arthritics go through the aspirin stage. The salicylate drug in aspirin can cause a very slight stimulation of the adrenal glands, which may provide an iota of relief. This has been reported in medical papers. The results, however, are not permanent.

In the majority of arthritics, pain may be the result of cartilage wearing out. These cartilages have no blood supply and cannot be regenerated. Aspirin can <u>not</u> repair the cartilage or the linings of our joints.

Nevertheless, some people take two, four, ten, or twenty-four aspirins a day. Pain may ease, but it is only a temporary measure. There is not one solitary particle of oil in 24 or 2,400 aspirin tablets. There is not an aspirin in the world that will make <u>lubricating oil</u> for your joint cavities!

X-Ray and Heat Treatments

There is no doubt that X-ray, diathermy, and ultra-violet rays are somewhat beneficial in treating arthritis of the hip and spine. This is known as the baking treatment. When pain goes beyond the aspirin stage, someone may turn the heat on you. Before heat is applied, though, a careful investigation of the patient's eating habits should be made. Because this kind of treatment, to be successful, must have help from your diet.

Any radiologist, orthopedist or X-ray technician who employs heat therapy should first check the patient's diet. Several weeks before undergoing any "baking," arthritics need daily intake of cod liver oil to give these powerful rays something to work on. X-rays bleed oil from tissues and they require added oil from the diet.

In physical medicine departments of hospitals and clinics, deformed arthritics sometimes go through another form of heat treatment. The paraffin-wax routine. Any arthritic who does not also change his dietary habits before undergoing this "wax bath" is wasting his time. Paraffin-wax heat in itself does not restore vitality to the blood vessels. This type of therapy, we predict, will decline in the years to come.

Frequently, after an arthritic has been subjected to hit-and-miss heat techniques for a long period of time, the whirlpool is suggested. Again, no appreciable improvement will be registered without a change of diet.

Gold Salts Are a Waste of Time

With all our education, how can we possibly think of gold salts as ever curing arthritis? The joint lining is not made up of gold. Neither is the joint's lubricating oil. The joint capsule, bursae, ligaments, etc., are not metal waiting for another metal to be pounded into them like someone building a skyscraper. The irritation to our sensitive bodies is terrific! How many failures do the gold salt manufacturers have to experience before they give up?

Yet, as fast as a hundred doctors have given up gold treatment, another hundred begin trying it out. Once and for all, there is no magic cure in gold salts for arthritis.

Penicillin Can't Help

No specific germ has ever been isolated that is responsible for either osteo or rheumatoid arthritis. So, unfortunately, the popular germ-killer known as penicillin is of no aid to arthritis.

In penicillin there is not one drop of oil to arrest a squeaking joint. It would be wonderful if arthritics could walk into a doctor's office, receive a beneficial injection of 100,000 units of penicillin, and stay cured, but it's impossible. With penicillin, or any other anti-biotic on the market today.

There are, and probably always will be, a few doctors who will try injecting vaccine. The vaccines themselves are of two kinds, autogenous and stock synthesized. Autogenous means self-originating. Autogenous vaccines are vaccines made from bacteria already inside the patient's body during fevers or inflammation. Stock vaccines are created in laboratory test-tubes. The theory is that if you inject bacteria from one disease (like typhoid) and cause an abnormally high fever, when the fever recedes it may take away your arthritis, too.

Doctors begin by giving small doses of ten million micro-organisms, then lead up to two billion organisms. A violent body reaction results. Some of the better known vaccines are Coley's, Crome's typhoid, a non-specific protein vaccine like sulphur, and a bee-venom preparation named apiolan. Even the doctors who used vaccine therapy soon saw its limitations. The fever caused was sometimes worse than the arthritis.

Still another injection experiment involved arsenic salts. Today we hear little of arsenic being used as a drug in the treatment of arthritis. Yet, because a limited number of arthritics thought they felt better temporarily, arsenic was known and used for a time as a blood stimulator. We could delve into a dozen other drugs like strychnine, quinine, nitrates and bromides. All have been tried out on the arthritic and all have failed.

Thyroid Extracts Have Some Merit

Doctors treating arthritis next turned to compounds derived from thyroid extracts. We believe these preparations may do you some good, because of the iodine value. Sixty per cent of your body's iodine is tied up in the thyroid gland. When you lack vigor, a basal metabolism test will generally reveal a sluggish thyroid. A good percentage of osteo and rheumatoid arthritics have a sluggish thyroid gland.

Such a thyroid deficiency usually indicates a lack of body iodine. Symptoms of this deficiency include dry skin, brittle nails and slow pulse. Also, you may notice coarser skin over the ankles, cheek bones, and back of the hands, or intermittent swelling about the eyes, cold and clammy legs or hands.

To correct these conditions, however, instead of taking a thyroid extract (a compound like potassium iodide) why not use simple cod liver oil? The iodine in cod liver oil can nourish an ailing thyroid —plus the entire arthritic body! The arthritic choosing cod liver oil for its iodine can easily correct his many external symptoms of dryness. And, at the very same time, he will be lubricating the joints themselves.

Do Diseased Organs Cause Arthritis?

Any doctor noticing inflamed tonsils, decayed teeth, or an irritated appendix, for example, will order surgical removal at once. That's fine, for your general health. But remember, diseased organs are not the cause of your arthritis. Originally, for some years, it was felt that fluids from infected organs traveled to your joints and made you arthritic. Later tests proved that there was no truth in this theory. A bad appendix or other ailing part will not create arthritis elsewhere in your body.

Surgery To Relieve Arthritic Pains

We have just explained that surgical operations on organs or glands cannot solve the question of arthritis. But can a doctor "operate" on actual arthritic bones and relieve your pain? The answer is "Yes."

After deformity has set in, there are a number of orthopedic operations which are helpful. More surgery will undoubtedly be devised in the future. Meanwhile, some of the operations now being used successfully for deformed arthritics only are known as synovectomy, arthrodesis, arthroplasty, etc.

Operations can be performed to remove any flesh-like tabs clinging to joint linings. These are frequently found in osteo arthritis, and sometimes they impede joint mobility. Surgery can also cut away some bone-spurs or extraneous deposits of cartilage or bone called "joint mice."

But before allowing your arthritis to reach the stage where surgical help is needed, wouldn't it be far better to practice the dietary and oil regime in this book? Prevent deformity by sane eating habits, and escape the surgeon's knife.

If a knee swells up to twice its normal size, and the trouble is a diseased lining, it is true that the joint membrane can be removed surgically. Joint linings will then regenerate, and your body will build new ones. At that time you may decide to straighten out your diet, to protect your "second set" of linings. Why not eat correctly, now? You'll save yourself a trip to the surgeon and a long convalescence.

One type of deformity is "fusion." When a joint becomes fused, it is said to be ankylosed. An ankylosed joint is frequently free from pain. The operation known as arthrodesis is primarily designed to give the fused joint some degree of service . . at least enable it to bear some weight. An arthroplasty operation will improve ball and socket joint mobility, by inserting a metal cup in your joint. Again, we say, however, stop your arthritic advancement by diet, before you need to undergo these major measures.

A Complete Physical Examination for Arthritics

As we near the end of this book, we are discovering that one key factor has been missing in the treatment of arthritics. In too many cases, a person with arthritis has never had a complete physical examination.

You may doubt that statement, and say that you have often been examined thoroughly from head to toe at your doctor's office. True, but what questions were you asked? Did anyone take a record of your past diet? Did the subject of cod liver oil come up in the discussion? Were tests made to determine the oil content of your body and of the foods you had been eating recently.

The point we are making is that most examinations for arthritis do not go far enough. They do not probe deeply enough into your background and eating habits—as well as the physical structure and condition of your body.

How can you be expected to become well, if you never really learn the full extent of your arthritis and the mistakes you are making to prolong the disease? Therefore, as a final aid to arthritics, we shall now give you a guide on how to obtain a complete physical examination the next time you visit your doctor. Here are the areas he should examine and the questions you should discuss together.

From Head To Foot, a Check List on Arthritis . . .

The extent and seriousness of your arthritic condition must be determined by starting to look for symptoms in your **HAIR** and **SCALP.** Is your hair lustrous? Does it fall out easily? Review your diet to see if it includes germinating foods. Does your diet include raw wheat germ, raw onion, garlic, scallion, and the jackets of baked potatoes— foods which can check an abnormal rate of hair loss.

Are either the hair or the scalp dry? If so, is there enough butter in your diet, and other oils?

Check the color of the hair. If it is greying too quickly, how much citrus juice have you consumed through the years? Curb them. These juices and fruits are too strong for most people. In most instances, color of hair is not determined by age, but by diet.

THE EARS should be examined with an oto-scope, an ear mirror, to record the amount of ear-wax. If there is wax present, what color is it? What consistency? What quantity? If none is present, is the ear itchy? How long has the ear been dry? Dry ears are serious indications of a dietary deficiency. Everyone should have ear wax all the time.

THE EYES should be studied, especially their corners and borders. When you wake up, do you have encrustations in the corners of your eyes? Do the conjunctivae look dry? Are glasses worn? If you are near-sighted, what quantities of fruit juice or carbonated soda pop did you consume during childhood? These liquids produce carbonic acid in the system, a condition detrimental to your eyes.

YOUR NOSE may be "itchy." If so, how long has it been that way? Do you have blackheads? Does too much sugar in your diet cause them? How much sugar have you been putting on cereal all these years? Correct or modify your sugar intake.

THE TEETH should be checked. There is no such thing as having an "average" number of cavities per month. If several cavities appear every six months, this is a definite indication that your diet is faulty. Incidentally, the fluorine in cod liver oil will help harden your teeth.

THE NECK can show symptoms, too. Look for wrinkles in the skin, on the sides and back of the neck. If they are there, you may have very little elasticity in your tissues. A leathery neck, loss of elasticity, come from too much sun. These warnings are also signs of a dangerous diet.

THE SKIN AND COMPLEXION deserve special attention. Are there any whitish-looking or scaly areas over the ankles, elbows, or knees? Does your skin have a natural shine to it? Are any skin creams or lotions applied? If so, when did you start using them? Perhaps this would give an approximate indication as to when the diet went wrong. Instead of externally applied oil to defeat dryness, you need dietary oils inside your body.

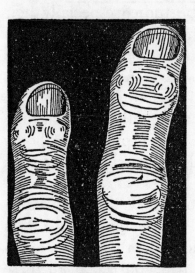

TYPICAL OF ARTHRITIS IN THE FINGERS. . . . Splitting nails with ridges, that break easily . . . swollen and stiffened joints.

FINGERNAILS take their nourishment from our blood. They depend on oils from the bloodstream. Are your nails brittle? Do they have ridges? Do they split easily? Cod liver oil will help check these conditions.

YOUR VEINS offer tell-tale signs, too. Look for varicose veins in the calves of your legs. Their presence indicates poor eating habits.

THE RECTAL AREA needs to be investigated. Is there an itching near the lower spine? If so, this is an early warning in many cases that your spinal vertebrae are going to have future trouble. It is quite possible that the oils near the lower vertebrae are drying out. You are being alerted by this sign that in five to ten years you may expect serious back ailments to set in.

MENTAL ATTITUDES can affect arthritis. Wise counsel by your own doctor can help set your mind at ease on most problems. You do <u>not</u> need a psychiatrist.

Some doctors may turn to psychosomatic medicine, but few arthritics need a full treatment by a specialist in psychiatry. It has been proven, though, that mental upset can hinder your recovery from arthritis. Dr. Hans Seyle of Montreal, Canada, wrote a complete report on this theory. What actually happens, among other things, is that too much worry interferes with the body's ability to produce its natural cortisone.

Medical Tests You Should Expect To Take

We have been discussing the various symptoms and external bodily signs which your doctor should check when examining you for arthritis. We have listed some of the questions he should ask, and we have even mentioned how your mind plays a part.

In addition to all of the above steps, your doctor may want to be even more thorough and make several other types of tests. Often, it is advisable to have blood chemistry reports on blood sugar levels, calcium, uric acid, phosphorus, cholesterol and protein, plus a test on liver functions and a complete urinalysis.

Naturally, blood pressure will be recorded and there will probably be a basal metabolism done.

All we are asking the medical profession to do —for your benefit—is to examine arthritics in connection with their diet. Continue all the present tests and examinations, but include dietary investigations, too!

The day is fast approaching when temporary aid will be given the rheumatoid arthritic through means of cortisone. And as soon as cortisone has started the patient on the road to recovery, then the dietary measures in this book will be prescribed— to maintain the improvement.

For osteo arthritis and many other rheumatic conditions, the diets and cod liver oil regime in this book are better than any other known approach.

HELP YOURSELF TO HEALTH

Each arthritic who will carry out the rules and regulations of self-examination and self-dieting can help himself. And you will need fewer trips to the doctor.

Just follow the dietary procedure and the common sense suggestions in this book. These discoveries are safe, sane and sound.

Doctors are busy with the many advanced arthritics who need their time. Medical men should be pleased to be free from arthritics who can correct their own individual dieting and bad eating habits.

May I repeat—I have always recommended that people who are ill should visit their doctors first. Your own physician is the man to see, to determine whether you have arthritis. Consult your doctor for a diagnosis, and return to him for periodic check-ups to chart the progress of your recovery.

This book does maintain, however, that it is possible for you to gain relief right in your own home. Through practicing simple diet controls.

Arthritis is an age-old curse, but now it can be corrected.

Proper diet and the use of cod liver oil are the keys to better health for millions of arthritics. This book has given you the facts. Your chance to gain relief from arthritis is now up to you. Apply the dietary program explained in these pages. You will be fighting arthritis with my proven discoveries . and with your own common sense.

Send a Copy of This Book to a Friend

All of us know many people who have arthritis. Perhaps you have a relative or a friend who is afflicted with this disease. Someone who would really appreciate receiving a copy of this book. Why not send a copy of "Arthritis and Common Sense" as a gift? It's a sensible gesture . . . you may be giving good health to a person who suffers from arthritis. They'll be grateful to you for years to come.

This page is to tell you how you can obtain another copy of this book. Bookstores often may not be able to keep enough copies in stock. Try your local book department, first. Or, if you wish, you can write directly to the publishers and they will immediately mail you as many copies as you need.